GUIDANCE DOCUMENT

I0482703

Administrating the Alaska Native Adult Tobacco Survey

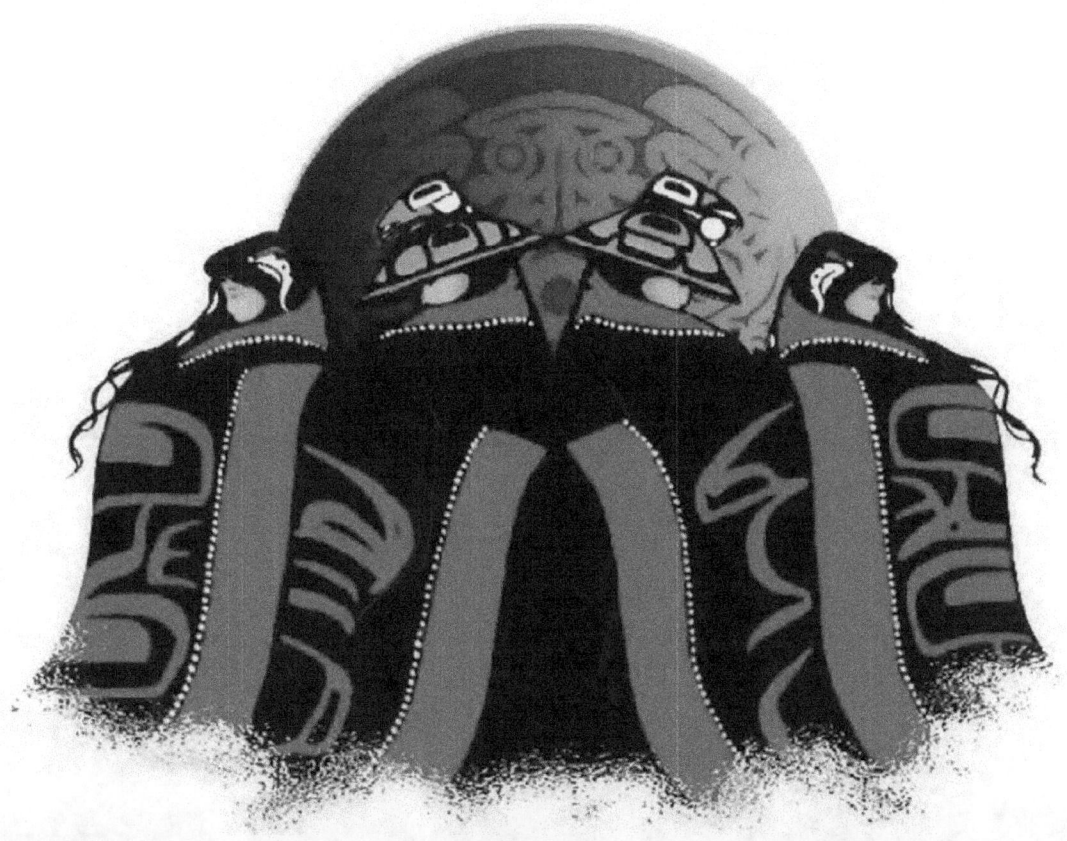

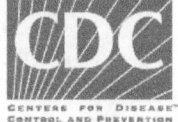

Guidance Document for Administrating the Alaska Native Adult Tobacco Survey

Art for front cover: Sierra Gerlach, Health Education and Promotion Council, Inc., 2433 W. Chicago, Suite C, Rapid City, SD 57702

Authors:

Victoria A. Albright, MA[1]

Sara Mirza, MPH[2]

Ralph S. Caraballo, PhD, MPH[2]

Adriane Niare, MPH, CHES[2]

Stacy L. Thorne, PhD, MPH, CHES[2]

[1] RTI International

[2] Centers for Disease Control and Prevention, National Center of Chronic Disease Prevention and Health Promotion, Office on Smoking and Health, Epidemiology Branch

Acknowledgments:

Alaska Native Health Board, Anchorage, AK

Alaska Native Tribal Health Consortium, Anchorage, AK

Alaska Native Adult Tobacco Survey Coordinator: St. Paul and Unalaska, AK

Alaska Native Adult Tobacco Survey Interviewers: St. Paul and Unalaska, AK

Alaska Native Adult Tobacco Survey Participants: St. Paul and Unalaska, AK

Arctic Slope Native Corporation, Barrow, AK

Maniilaq Health Center, Kotzebue, AK

Norton Sound Health Corporation, Nome, AK

Rita Anniskett

Daria Dirks

Alyssa Easton, PhD, MPH

Jenny Jennings Foerst, PhD

Andrea Fenaughty, PhD

Nick Gonzales

Charlotte Gisvold

Corrine Husten, MD, MPH

Doreen O. Lacy

Brick Lancaster, MA, CHES

Barbara Parks, RDH, MPH

Jay Macedo, MA

Brenna Muldavin, MS

Trena Rairdon

Loreano Reano, MPA

Laura Revels

Caroline C Renner

Cynthia Tainpeah, RN

Ray Tainpeah, MEd, LADC

Janis Weber, PhD

Suggested citation:

Albright VA, Mirza S, Caraballo R, Niare A, Thorne SL. Guidance document for administrating the Alaska Native Adult Tobacco Survey. U.S. Department of Health and Human Services, Centers for Disease Control and Prevention; 2010.

RTI International is a trade name of Research Triangle Institute.

Guidance Document for Administering the Alaska Adult Tobacco Survey

Contents

Tables

Figure

1. INTRODUCTION

The Centers for Disease Control and Prevention (CDC) and health care professionals across the State of Alaska share a vision, a mission, and specific goals for improving the health and well-being of Alaska Natives.

Vision. The shared vision is for all Alaska Natives to live healthy, tobacco-free lives.

Mission. The shared mission is to provide leadership, coordinate resources, and promote efforts that support Alaska Natives in living healthy, tobacco-free lives.

Goals. The specific goals to promote this vision and mission are

- to eliminate exposure to secondhand tobacco smoke,

- to identify and eliminate disparities between population groups with regard to attitudes toward, knowledge about, and use of tobacco,

- to promote the quitting of tobacco use among adults and youth, and

- to prevent initiation of tobacco use among youth and young adults.

CDC offers this guidance document to support users of the Alaska Native Adult Tobacco Survey (AN ATS).

1.1   Smoking and Health Among Alaska Natives

A direct relation exists between a population's health and its use of tobacco (American Nonsmokers' Rights Foundation, 2010b; Centers for Disease Control and Prevention, 2004). Scientific studies have shown that tobacco use causes various cancers, respiratory and cardiovascular diseases, and adverse pregnancy outcomes. Because of these multiple detriments to health, tobacco use remains the leading cause of preventable death in Alaska, with more deaths occurring from tobacco use than from motor vehicle crashes, suicides, homicides, and air transport crashes combined (Alaska Department of Health and Social Services, 2006).

Existing surveillance data suggest that Alaska Natives' rate of tobacco use is especially high. The leading cause of death for Alaska Natives is cancer; moreover, lung cancer, which is caused primarily by smoking tobacco, is for this population the leading cause of cancer death. In fact, tobacco use causes one of every three cancer deaths among Alaska Natives. In addition to causing high rates of cancer, the high rates of tobacco use among Alaska Natives may translate into cardiovascular disease and chronic obstructive pulmonary disease; for Alaska Native children, exposure to secondhand smoke may mean more cases of asthma, bronchitis, pneumonia, and sudden infant death syndrome (Alaska Department of Health and Social Services, 2006).

As noted therein, state and local initiatives in Alaska have sought to reduce tobacco use and reduce the health risks for Alaskans. These efforts have helped many people, and important progress has been made. For example, since 1993 cigarette smoking among youth in Alaska has dramatically decreased. Nevertheless, much more work remains to be done.

1.2 The Alaska Native Adult Tobacco Survey Guidance Document

This AN ATS guidance document was developed by CDC, Office on Smoking and Health (OSH), for health professionals who plan to implement the AN ATS in Alaska Native villages and communities. Many methods and strategies delineated here are drawn from CDC's experience fielding the AN ATS in Alaska and are fundamental to conducting an efficient, scientifically rigorous survey.

The guidelines are organized under nine main headings:

1. Introduction

2. Survey Instruments and Supporting Materials

3. Survey Planning and Budgeting

4. Sampling and Weighting

5. Interviewer Training

6. Enhancing Response Rates

7. Data Preparation

8. Analysis and Reporting

9. References and Resources

Information on CDC's broad-based efforts to help reduce tobacco use can be found at http://www.cdc.go. Readers may contact CDC/OSH by e-mail at tobaccoinfo@cdc.gov or by phone at 1-800-CDC-INFO. Readers may visit the OSH Online Publications Catalog at http://www.cdc.gov/tobacco/publications/index.htm to order OSH publications and materials.

The AN ATS instruments and survey materials were approved by the Office of Management and Budget for use in two CDC-supported surveys in Alaska.

1.3   The Role of Alaska Native Adult Tobacco Survey Findings in Future Program Design and Evaluation

Surveillance data on tobacco use are an essential evaluation tool and can aide in building effective programs to reduce smoking and secondhand exposure to tobacco smoke. For Alaska Natives, such data have been limited, especially at the community level. The AN ATS was developed to collect data specifically from Alaska Native persons in order that tribal health officials may set health priorities and develop approaches for reducing tobacco use while being respectful of Alaska Natives' culture (Alaska Department of Health and Social Services, 2007). The survey can be used by future programs that focus on decreasing Alaska Natives' tobacco burden.

The AN ATS elicits information on the following topics:

- prevalence rates of commercial cigarette smoking among members of the community

- use of other tobacco products (i.e., iqmik, chewing or "spit" tobacco, and snuff or dip tobacco)

- efforts and methods used to quit using tobacco

- readiness to quit using tobacco

- physicians' and health professionals' advice about quitting

- secondhand smoke exposure

- workplace policies on smoking

- risk perception and tobacco-related knowledge, attitudes, and opinions

- demographic information

Findings from the AN ATS will enhance understanding of the extent of tobacco use among Alaska Native men and women older than age 18. Questions about smoking behaviors that occurred before this age will lend insight into practices among younger people. Once the data are collected and analyzed, interventions can be implanted on the basis of these findings.

Measures of tobacco-related knowledge, attitudes, and opinions are used to gain an understanding of smokers' readiness to change and are used to gain an appreciation of the barriers to quitting and reasons for relapsing. The knowledge, attitudes, and opinions information collected with the AN ATS can be used to develop intervention strategies. Incorporating such information into programs has been shown to effect positive changes in smoking behaviors (Horwath, 1999; Prochaska et al., 1994). Prevention and cessation interventions and programs can be targeted, for example, to the specific segments of the

Alaska Native population most injured by tobacco use or exposure to tobacco smoke, or can be targeted to youth to reduce the number who start smoking.

In addition to informing new programs, The AN ATS findings can help communities evaluate the success of extant programs. Such evaluations can be used to refine intervention strategies or suggest alternative ones. AN ATS data may be included, moreover, in funding and grant applications to support these programs.

1.4   The Alaska Native Adult Tobacco Survey Questionnaire

The AN ATS is a comprehensive tobacco survey that addresses the goals, mission, and objectives of the health community. The questions were cognitively tested with all five major Alaska Native ethnic groups (Aleut, Athabascan, Inupiat, Yupik, and Alitiiq) to ensure cultural sensitivity to and appropriateness for Alaska Natives. The questions and vocabulary reflect the experience and language of Alaska Natives; the reading comprehension level facilitates understanding by participants with various degrees of literacy. The questions were administered in English because the vast majority of Alaska Natives speak English. Skip patterns were integrated to help participants move through the survey efficiently.

Two versions of the questionnaire are available. They collect the same survey information but take into account different sampling methods. One version—called the *Member List Version*—is designed for use with a shareholder list or other comparable sampling frame of individual, eligible Alaska Native adults from which a random sample has been drawn. If, instead, a sample of households has been drawn, the *Household List Version* should be used in conjunction with the AN ATS Household Screener. This screener is administered to any adult member of the household in order to (1) establish whether any Alaska Natives reside in the household and, if so, (2) select one Alaska Native household member at random to complete the survey.

The AN ATS questionnaires, survey supporting materials, and other resources are available as the following appendices:

A. Advance Letter

B. Household Screener

C. Informed Consent

D. Readability of the Informed Consent Form

E. "Sorry I Missed You" Card

F. Receipt

G. Cognitive Evaluation Highlights

H. Letter to Request Permission or Engage Cooperation of the Tribal Organization

I. Interviewer Training Manual

J. Survey (Household List Version)

K. Survey (Member List Version)

1.5 The Goal of Data Quality

The goal of the AN ATS and this guidance document is to help the Alaskan health care community gather information that is meaningful, complete, reliable, valid, precise, and unbiased. The methods and approaches described here are designed to maximize data quality by reducing the possibility that errors will be made in

- questions asked,

- people selected to respond,

- data collection,

- data processing, or

- statistical analysis.

High-data quality will help ensure that the findings from the AN ATS are credible and that the decisions and programs based on these data will be appropriate for the particular service area.

A description of all the various kinds of errors that can occur in survey research is beyond the scope of this guidance document. For more information on this topic, see the references and resources provided in Chapter 9.

2. SURVEY INSTRUMENTS AND SUPPORTING MATERIALS

This chapter provides information on the Alaska Native Adult Tobacco Survey (AN ATS) questionnaire and offers guidance on survey administration. Interviewers will find this information helpful before they administer questions; analysts will find it helpful for interpreting results.

2.1 Topics Covered in the Alaska Native Adult Tobacco Survey

The AN ATS provides a core set of tobacco-related questions, demographic items, and the opportunity to add questions of local relevance. The AN ATS was modeled on the General Population State ATS and other well-established tobacco-use surveys. Because AN ATS users may want to compare their findings with those of other ATS surveys, a crucial construct to consider in all tobacco-use surveys is the definition of *smoker*. The AN ATS enables its users to define smokers exactly as smokers are defined in most major national and state-level tobacco-use surveys.

In the design of the AN ATS, seven topics were identified as the most central and critical to health programs among Alaska Natives; the AN ATS provides a battery of questions, referred to as *core questions,* relevant to these topics:

- general health

- cigarette smoking and quitting

- iqmik use and quitting

- chewing (spit) tobacco use and quitting

- snuff or dip tobacco use and quitting

- secondhand smoke exposure

- perception of risks related to tobacco use

To the greatest extent possible, the precise questions used in the AN ATS were drawn from or based on previously tested and validated surveys. Some questions were added and others were modified to suit the specific circumstances and culture of Alaska Natives. The questions were organized by topic and sequenced logically for ease of administration. Questionnaire drafts were tested with representative participants and from five Alaska Native tribes and further modified in response to participants' comments.

The AN ATS is administered to adults aged 18 years or older. To elicit information about the behaviors of youth, the questionnaire asks these adult participants about their tobacco use before age 18. All survey participants are asked at least some questions on each core topic, except questions about quitting smoking are asked of current and former smokers only, not of those whose responses indicate that they have never smoked.

The AN ATS questionnaire includes a set of questions to collect demographic information. For the AN ATS Member List Version, these questions appear at the end of the Member List Version questionnaire; for the Household List Version, these items are divided between the AN ATS Household Screener and the end of the Household List Version questionnaire. Identical demographic questions are designated by identical item numbers, regardless of where they appear.

The AN ATS questionnaire is organized to allow special questions, referred to as *user-selected questions*, to be added to address issues of local concern.

2.2   Determining the Respondent's Smoking Status

Defining smokers' status is important also because it determines the path respondents (Rs) follow through the questionnaire. Rs can be either *current smokers* or *former smokers*, or they may be classified as *triers or experimenters* or as *never smokers*, according to the working definitions in the survey. This same classification of Rs by smoking status is used in the General Population State ATS.

Responses to three key questions to classify Rs' smoking status:

Q2:   Have you ever smoked a cigarette, even one or two puffs? Responses: "Yes," "No," "Don't know / Not sure," or "Refused."

Q4:   In your entire life, have you smoked at least 100 cigarettes, about five packs? Responses: "Yes," "No," "Don't know / not sure," or "Refused."

Q6:   Do you now smoke cigarettes every day, some days, or not at all? Responses: "Every day," "Some days," "Not at all," "Don't know / not sure," or "Refused."

Current smokers. In most adult surveys, a *current smoker* is a defined as an R who has smoked at least 100 cigarettes in his or her lifetime and was smoking every day or some days at the time of survey. The R will have answered "Yes" to Q2, "Yes" to Q4, and "Every day" or "Some days" to Q6.

Former smokers. A *former smoker* is an R who has smoked at least 100 cigarettes during his or her lifetime and currently does not smoke. The R will have answered "Yes" to Q2, "Yes" to Q4, and "Not at all" to Q6.

Never smokers. The R is classified as never having smoked if the R says he or she has not smoked at least 100 cigarettes during his or her lifetime. The R will have answered "Yes or No" to Q2 and "No" to Q4.

Triers or experimenters. The R is classified as a *trier,* or *experimenter,* if he or she answered "Yes" to Q2 and "No" to Q4.

Questions about iqmik use, chewing tobacco, and snuff tobacco are included in the AN ATS. Iqmik use and chewing and snuff tobacco are common in Alaska Native populations and of interest to public health practitioners in Alaska Native communities.

2.3 Question-by-Question Guidance

2.3.1 Section 1: Introduction

In order to assess the comprehensibility of the survey questions for Alaska Natives, the AN ATS was subjected to thorough testing with representative survey participants. The testing identified terms possibly confusing for the Rs, or ones that may benefit from clarification. In addition, the testing helped identify effective ways for the interviewer to probe ambiguous or unclear responses.

Interviewers should review this question-by-question information and use the suggested clarifications and probes when administering the AN ATS. Doing so will produce higher-quality data. This information may also help analysts to interpret data because they will understand how Rs interpret the questions.

2.3.2 Section 2: General Health

The General Health section (Q1) consists of a single question asking the R to give his or her subjective evaluation of his or her general health.

Q1:   ***General health status.*** In the cognitive interviews, Rs generally avoided selecting the top two response options for this question. Rs who felt physically well but had been some time without a physician's examination were reluctant to choose these responses, because they could not be sure nothing was wrong with their health. The same was true for those who felt very well but knew they had not followed a healthy lifestyle (e.g., smokers or those who did not exercise).

2.3.3 Section 3: Cigarette Smoking

The 11 questions about cigarette smoking (Q2 to Q12) elicit information about the R's lifetime and current cigarette smoking. Rs are asked if they have ever smoked a cigarette in their lifetime and, if so, at what age they first smoked. Current smokers and former smokers are asked what their age was when they began smoking regularly. Rs who have smoked are asked if they have smoked at least 100 cigarettes in their lives. Rs who report smoking in the past 30 days are asked how many days they have smoked in the past 30, how many cigarettes they have smoked per day, how soon they first smoke after waking, and what their most frequently smoked brand is.

Questions about the age at which the R first smoked and the age at which the R began regularly smoking provide important insight into smoking habits.

Q2:   ***Whether R has ever smoked a cigarette.*** This question asks the R if he has ever smoked a cigarette, even one or two puffs. The reference period is the R's entire life. All questions regarding cigarette smoking are about tobacco cigarettes only and do not include marijuana or any other smoked substances rolled in paper.

Q3: ***Age at R's first time smoking.*** This question is asked only of those who answered "Yes" in Q2. Responses must be in years of age. Responses such as "5 years ago" or "in my last year of high school" should be probed for exact age.

Q4: ***Whether R has smoked at least 100 cigarettes in his or her lifetime.*** This question is intended to elicit whether the R has smoked a total of 100 cigarettes in his or her lifetime, not in a single day. In testing it appeared that smokers were accustomed to reporting daily cigarette consumption and tended to hear this question as asking about a single day. The interviewer should stress "not on a single day." Training should focus on this issue because this question is key to determining the R's smoking status. As applies to any question, if an R says something that suggests he or she has misunderstood the question, the interviewer should repeat the question or that part of it that has been misunderstood.

Q5: ***Age at which R started smoking regularly.*** This question is intended to determine the age at which R began smoking *regularly*, not age of initiation. Interviewer should stress the word *regularly*. No definition of *regularly* is provided to R. The interviewer must ensure that R provides an actual number for age, rather than a description such as "in high school."

Q6: ***Whether R currently smokes every day, some days, or not at all.*** The reference period for this question is the present, without further definition. This question elicits current smoking status and is used to identify the category of "current smokers," "former smokers," "triers or experimenters," and "never smokers."

Q7: ***Days R smoked in the past 30.*** The reference period is the 30 days before the interview date. Responses not provided in number of days (responses given as frequency—e.g., "every day" or "twice a week") should be probed, with stress on "how many days."

Q8: ***Cigarettes smoked per day on days when R smoked in the past 30.*** The reference period is the 30 days before the interview date. The question is intended to elicit average daily consumption on days when R smoked. In cognitive testing, some Rs answered in ways that may pose calculation problems for the interviewers. Interviewers should practice probing or coding answers such as "I smoke a pack in 3 days" or "I smoke two packs in a day and a half."

Q9: ***How soon after waking R smokes the first cigarette.*** This question offers categories to elicit the time elapsed between R's waking and the first cigarette smoking of the day. The question indicates that the response options must be read aloud to the R. Some Rs associate smoking with specific activities and may first answer in that way (e.g., "I light up right after breakfast"). Such uncodable responses should be probed; the response categories, repeated.

Q10: ***Brand R most frequently smokes.*** The list of cigarette brands offered includes generic (or no-brand) cigarettes.

Q11: ***Whether R had access to a computer in the past 12 months.*** The reference period is the 12 months before the interview date.

Q12: ***Whether R bought cigarettes on the Internet.*** The reference period is the 12 months before the interview date.

Attempts to Quit Smoking

Two questions (Q13 and Q14) address attempts to quit smoking. These questions are asked of "current smokers."

Q13: ***Time elapsed since R last smoked a cigarette.*** This item provides additional information about the category of smoker that best fits R: "current smoker," "former smoker," "trier or experimenter," or "never smoker."

Q14: ***Quit attempts lasting longer than 1 day.*** It is important to ensure that R listens to this entire question before answering; otherwise, he or she may answer "Yes" for reasons other than quitting smoking for a day or longer because he or she was trying to quit (e.g., if R was in the hospital for a day or longer).

Methods of Quitting (Smoking)

Six questions (Q15 to Q20) address methods of quitting smoking, including nontraditional methods of quitting (Q19). These questions are asked of "current smokers" and "former smokers."

Q15–18: ***Medications used to assist in quitting; "cold turkey" quitting.*** These questions are asked only of "current smokers" or "former smokers" who quit during the 5 years preceding the interview.

Q19: ***Use of prayer or pledge to assist in quitting.*** This question is asked only of "current smokers" or "former smokers" who quit during the 5 years preceding the interview.

Q20: ***Use of classes or counseling to assist in quitting.*** This question is asked only of "current smokers" who made a quit attempt in the past year or of "former smokers" who quit in the past 5 years. Alternate introductions are provided for the two types of R.

Readiness to Quit Smoking

Three questions (Q21 to Q23) address stages of change for quitting. These questions are asked of "current smokers" only.

Q21–23: ***Readiness of R to quit smoking.*** These questions are asked only of "current smokers." An R who smokes only some days may not feel these questions are relevant. The interviewer should ask the R to answer the questions as accurately and completely as possible.

Physicians' and Health Professionals' Advice to Quit Smoking

There are 11 questions (Q24 to Q27h) that address physicians' and health professionals' advice.

Q24: ***Receipt of health checkup or care in the past 12 months.*** Both "current smokers" and "former smokers" who quit smoking during the 5 years preceding the interview answer this item.

Q25:   ***Health professional's asking whether R smokes.*** This question is asked only of Rs who have seen a health professional during the 12 months preceding the interview ("yes" at Q24).

Q26:   ***Health professional's advice not to smoke.*** This and subsequent items in this section are asked only of Rs who answered "yes" at Q24.

Q27a–h: ***Health professional's recommendation to use quit aids.*** This sequence is asked of any R whose health care professional either advised against smoking or asked R whether he smoked.

2.3.4 Section 4: Iqmik Use

The 10 questions about iqmik use (Q28 to Q37) elicit information about the R's lifetime and current iqmik use. Q29 and Q31 are used to determine the iqmik use status of an R. More than 50% of Yupik people in the Yukon-Kuskokwim Delta still use iqmik. Among pregnant women, use rises to an alarming 80%. Users often reason that, because the ingredients are "all natural" (dried tobacco leaves and punk ash), iqmik is less harmful to a fetus than commercial tobacco products. However, iqmik delivers a powerful dose of poisoning to both mother and fetus. Health agencies are working hard to redirect this aspect of Yupik culture (Pleninger & Volk, 2005).

Rs are asked if they have ever used iqmik in their lifetime and, if so, at what age they first used iqmik. Rs who have used iqmik are asked if they have used iqmik at least 20 times in their lives. Rs who report using iqmik in the past 30 days are asked how many days they have used iqmik in the past 30, how many times they used per day, how soon they first used after waking, and where they obtain their iqmik.

Q28:   ***Lifetime use of iqmik.*** This question asks the R if he has ever used iqmik. The reference period is the R's entire life.

Q29:   ***Use of iqmik at least 20 times.*** This question is intended to elicit whether the R has used iqmik a total of 20 times in his or her lifetime, not in a single day. The interviewer should stress "in your entire life." As applies to any question, if an R says something that suggests he or she has misunderstood the question, the interviewer should repeat the question or that part of it that has been misunderstood.

Q30:   ***Regular use of iqmik.*** This question is intended to determine whether R has ever used iqmik regularly. Interviewer should stress the word *regularly*.

Q31:   ***Age at which R began using iqmik regularly.*** This question is intended to determine the age at which R began using iqmik *regularly*, not age of initiation. Interviewer should stress the word *regularly*. No definition of *regularly* is provided to R. The interviewer must ensure that R provides an actual number for the age, rather than a description such as "in high school."

Q32:   ***Regular use of iqmik currently.*** This question is intended to determine whether R is currently a regular user of iqmik.

Q33:   ***Daily use of iqmik.*** The reference period for this question is the present, without further definition. This question elicits current iqmik use status and is used to identify the category of "current iqmik users."

Q34: ***Use of iqmik in the past 30 days.*** The reference period is the 30 days before the interview date. Responses not provided in number of days (responses given as frequency—e.g., "every day" or "twice a week") should be probed, with stress on "how many days."

Q35: ***Times iqmik was used per day in the past 30 days.*** The reference period is the 30 days before the interview date. The question is intended to elicit average daily consumption on days when R used iqmik. In cognitive testing, some Rs answered in ways that may pose calculation problems for the interviewers.

Q36: ***Where iqmik is obtained.*** This question is used to determine the source of the iqmik.

Q37: ***How soon after waking R first uses iqmik.*** This question offers categories to elicit the time elapsed between R's waking and the first iqmik use of the day. The question indicates that the response options must be read aloud to the R. Some Rs associate iqmik use with specific activities and may first answer in that way (e.g., "I use iqmik right after breakfast"). Such uncodable responses should be probed; the response categories, repeated.

Attempts to Quit Iqmik Use

Two questions (Q38 to Q39) address attempts to quit using iqmik. These questions are asked of "current iqmik users."

Q38: ***Elapsed time since last iqmik use.*** It is important to read the response categories for this question to R. In cognitive testing, when response options were not explicitly offered, Rs gave complex answers that would be difficult for interviewers to code. Time references given in parentheses in the questionnaire are for interviewers to use at their discretion, to aid processing of R's answer or to probe an unclear response.

Q39: ***Iqmik quit attempts lasting longer than 1 day.*** It is important to ensure that R listens to the entire question before answering; otherwise, he or she may answer "yes" for reasons other than quitting iqmik use for a day or longer (e.g., if R was in the hospital for a day or longer).

Methods of Quitting (Iqmik)

Six questions (Q40 to Q45) address methods of quitting iqmik use, including nontraditional methods of quitting (Q44). These questions are asked of "current iqmik users" and "former iqmik users." Alternate introductions are provided for the two types of R.

Q40–43: ***Medications used to assist in quitting; "cold turkey" quitting.*** These questions are asked only of "current iqmik users" or "former iqmik users" who quit during the 5 years preceding the interview.

Q44: ***Use of prayer or pledge to assist in quitting.*** This question is asked only of "current iqmik users" or "former iqmik users" who quit during the 5 years preceding the interview.

Q45: ***Use of classes or counseling to assist in quitting.*** This question is asked only of "current iqmik users" who made a quit attempt in the year preceding the interview or of "former iqmik users" who quit during the 5 years preceding the interview.

Readiness to Quit Using Iqmik

Three questions (Q46 to Q48) address stages of change for quitting. These questions are asked of "current iqmik users" only.

Q46–48: ***Readiness to quit using iqmik.*** These questions are asked only of "current iqmik users."

Physicians' and Health Professionals' Advice to Quit Using Iqmik

Eleven questions (Q49 to Q52h) address physicians' and health professionals' advice.

Q49: ***Receipt of health checkup or care in the past 12 months.*** Both "current iqmik users" and "former iqmik users" who quit during the 5 years preceding the interview answer this question.

Q50: ***Health professional's asking whether R uses iqmik.*** This question is asked only of Rs who have seen a health professional during the 12 months preceding the interview ("yes" at Q49).

Q51: ***Health professional's advice not to use iqmik.*** This and subsequent items in this section are asked only of Rs who answered "yes" at Q49.

Q52a–h: ***Health professional's recommendation to use quit aids.*** This sequence is asked of any R whose health care professional either asked R whether he or she used iqmik, or advised against using iqmik.

2.3.5 Section 5: Chewing (Spit) Tobacco

The 12 questions about chewing or spit tobacco (Q53 to Q64) elicit information about the R's lifetime and current use of chewing tobacco. Q55 and Q57 are used to determine the chewing or spit tobacco use status of an R.

Rs are asked whether they have ever used chewing (or spit) tobacco in their lifetime and, if so, at what age they first used it. Rs who have used chewing tobacco are asked whether they have used chewing tobacco at least 20 times in their lives. Rs who report having used chewing tobacco during the 30 days preceding the interview are asked how many days they have used chewing tobacco in the past 30 days, how many times they have used chewing tobacco per day, how soon they first used chewing tobacco after waking, and where they obtain their chewing tobacco.

Q53: ***Lifetime use of chewing (or spit) tobacco.*** This question asks the R if he has ever used chewing or spit tobacco. The reference period is the R's entire life.

Q54: ***Use of chewing (or spit) tobacco at least 20 times.*** This question is intended to elicit whether the R has used chewing (or spit) tobacco at least 20 times in his or her lifetime, not in a single day. The interviewer should stress "in your entire life." As applies to any question, if an R says something that suggests he has misunderstood the question, the interviewer should repeat the question or that part of it that has been misunderstood.

Q55: ***Regular use of chewing (or spit) tobacco.*** This question is intended to determine whether R has ever used chewing or spit tobacco regularly. Interviewer should stress the word *regularly.*

Q56: ***Age at which R began using chewing (or spit) tobacco regularly.*** This question is intended to determine the age at which R began using chewing or spit tobacco *regularly*, not age of initiation. The interviewer should stress the word *regularly.* No definition of *regularly* is provided to R. The interviewer must ensure that R provides an actual number for the age, rather than a description such as "in high school."

Q57: ***Regular use of chewing (or spit) tobacco currently.*** This question is intended to determine whether R currently is a regular user of chewing (or spit) tobacco.

Q58: ***Daily use of chewing (or spit) tobacco.*** The reference period for this question is the present, without further definition. This question elicits current chewing tobacco-use status and is used to identify the category of "current chewing or spit tobacco users."

Q59: ***Use of chewing (or spit) tobacco in the past 30 days.*** The reference period is the 30 days preceding the interview. Responses not provided in number of days (responses given as frequency—e.g., "every day" or "twice a week") should be probed, with stress on "how many days."

Q60: ***Times per day chewing (or spit) tobacco was used in the past 30 days.*** The reference period is the 30 days preceding the interview. The question is intended to elicit average daily consumption on days when R used chewing tobacco. In cognitive testing, some Rs answered in ways that may pose calculation problems for the interviewers.

Q61: ***Where chewing (or spit) tobacco is obtained.*** This question is used to determine the source of the chewing tobacco.

Q62: ***How soon after waking R first uses chewing (or spit) tobacco.*** This question offers categories to elicit the time elapsed between R's waking and the first chewing tobacco use of the day. The question indicates that the response options must be read aloud to the R. Some Rs associate chewing tobacco use with specific activities and may first answer in that way (e.g., "I use chewing tobacco right after breakfast"). Such uncodable responses should be probed; the response categories, repeated.

Q63: ***Whether R had access to a computer.*** The reference period is the 12 months preceding the interview.

Q64: ***Whether R purchased chewing tobacco on the Internet.*** The reference period is the 12 months preceding the interview.

Attempts to Quit Chewing (or Spit) Tobacco

Two questions (Q65 to Q66) address attempts to quit using chewing (or spit) tobacco.

These questions are asked of "current chewing tobacco users."

Q65: ***Time elapsed since last use of chewing tobacco.*** It is important to read the response categories to R. In cognitive testing, when response options were not explicitly offered, Rs gave complex answers that would be difficult for interviewers to code. Time references given in parentheses in the questionnaire are for interviewers to use at their discretion, to aid processing of R's answer or to probe an unclear response.

Q66: ***Chewing tobacco quit attempts lasting longer than 1 day.*** It is important to ensure that R listens to this entire question before answering; otherwise, he or she may answer "Yes" for reasons other than quitting chewing tobacco for a day or longer (e.g., if R was in the hospital for a day or longer).

Methods of Quitting (Chewing or Spit Tobacco)

Six questions (Q67 to Q72) ask about methods of quitting chewing tobacco, including nontraditional methods of quitting (Q71). These questions are asked of "current chewing tobacco users" and "former chewing tobacco users." Alternate introductions are provided for the two types of R.

Q67–70: ***Medications used to assist in quitting; "cold turkey" quitting.*** These questions are asked only of "current chewing tobacco users" or "former chewing tobacco users" who quit during the 5 years preceding the interview.

Q71: ***Use of prayer or pledge to assist in quitting.*** This question is asked only of "current chewing tobacco users" or "former chewing tobacco users" who quit during the 5 years preceding the interview.

Q72: ***Use of classes or counseling to assist in quitting.*** This question is asked only of "current chewing tobacco users" who made a quit attempt in the year preceding the interview or of "former chewing tobacco users" who quit during the 5 years preceding the interview.

Readiness to Quit Chewing Tobacco

Three questions (Q73 to Q75) address stages of change for quitting. These questions are asked of "current chewing tobacco users" only.

Q73–75: ***Readiness to quit using chewing (or spit) tobacco.*** These questions are asked only of "current chewing tobacco users."

Physicians' and Health Professionals' Advice to Quit Chewing Tobacco

Eleven questions (Q76 to Q79h) address physicians' and health professionals' advice.

Q76: ***Receipt of health checkup or care in the past 12 months.*** Both "current chewing tobacco users" and "former chewing tobacco users" who quit during the 5 years preceding the interview answer this question.

Q77: ***Health professional's asking whether R uses chewing tobacco.*** This question is asked only of Rs who have seen a health professional in the 12 months preceding the interview ("yes" at Q76).

Q78: ***Health professional's advice not to use chewing tobacco.*** This and subsequent questions in this section are asked only of Rs who answered "yes" at Q76.

Q79a–h: ***Health professional's recommendation to use quit aids.*** This sequence is asked of any R whose health care professional either advised against using chewing tobacco or asked R whether he or she used chewing tobacco.

2.3.6 Section 6: Snuff or Dip Tobacco

Twelve questions about snuff or dip tobacco (Q80 to Q91) elicit information about the R's lifetime and current snuff or dip tobacco use. Q81 and Q83 are used to determine the snuff or dip tobacco-use status of an R.

Rs are asked if they have ever used snuff or dip tobacco in their lifetime and, if so, at what age they first used. Rs who have used snuff or dip tobacco are asked if they have used snuff or dip tobacco at least 20 times in their lives. Rs who report having used snuff or dip tobacco in the 30 days preceding the interview are asked how many days they have used snuff or dip tobacco in those 30 days, how many times they have used snuff or dip tobacco per day, how soon they first used snuff or dip tobacco after waking, and where they obtain their snuff or dip tobacco.

Q80:   ***Lifetime use of snuff or dip tobacco.*** This question asks the R if he or she has ever used snuff or dip tobacco. The reference period is the R's entire lifetime.

Q81:   ***Use of snuff or dip tobacco at least 20 times.*** This question is intended to elicit whether the R has used snuff or dip tobacco at least 20 times in his or her lifetime, not in a single day. The interviewer should stress "in your entire life." As applies to any question, if an R says something that suggests he or she has misunderstood the question, the interviewer should repeat the question or that part of it that has been misunderstood.

Q82:   ***Regular use of snuff or dip tobacco.*** This question is intended to determine whether R has ever used snuff or dip tobacco regularly. Interviewers should stress the word *regularly*.

Q83:   ***Age at which R first used snuff or dip tobacco regularly.*** This question is intended to determine the age at which R began using snuff or dip tobacco *regularly*, not age of initiation. Interviewer should stress the word *regularly*. No definition of what *regularly* means is provided to R. Interviewers must ensure that R provides an actual number for the age, rather than a description such as "in high school."

Q84:   ***Regular use of snuff or dip tobacco currently.*** This question is intended to determine whether R is currently a regular user of snuff or dip tobacco.

Q85:   ***Daily use of snuff or dip tobacco.*** The reference period for this question is the present, without further definition. This question elicits current snuff or dip tobacco-use status and is used to identify the category of "current snuff or dip tobacco users."

Q86:   ***Use of snuff or dip tobacco in the past 30 days.*** The reference period is the 30 days preceding the interview. Responses not provided in number of days (responses given as frequency—e.g., "every day" or "twice a week") should be probed, with stress on "how many days."

Q87:   ***Times per day snuff or dip tobacco was used in the past 30 days.*** The reference period is the 30 days preceding the interview. The question is intended to elicit average daily consumption on days when R used snuff or dip tobacco. In cognitive testing, some Rs answered in ways that may pose calculation problems for interviewers.

Q88: ***Where snuff or dip tobacco is obtained.*** This question is used to determine the source of the snuff or dip tobacco.

Q89: ***How soon after waking R first uses snuff or dip tobacco.*** This question offers categories to elicit the time elapsed between R's waking and the first snuff use of the day. The question indicates that the response options must be read aloud to the R. Some Rs associate snuff use with specific activities and may first answer in that way (e.g., "I use snuff right after breakfast"). Such uncodable responses should be probed; the response categories, repeated.

Q90: ***Whether R has access to a computer.*** The reference period is the 12 months preceding the interview.

Q91: ***Whether R purchased snuff or dip tobacco on the Internet.*** The reference period is the 12 months preceding the interview.

Attempts to Quit Snuff or Dip Tobacco

Two questions (Q92 to Q93) address attempts to quit using snuff or dip tobacco. These questions are asked of "current snuff or dip tobacco users."

Q92: ***Time elapsed since last use of snuff or dip tobacco.*** It is important to read the response categories for this question to R. In cognitive testing, when response options were not explicitly offered, Rs gave complex answers that would be difficult for interviewers to code. Time references given in parentheses are for interviewers to use at their discretion, to aid processing of R's answer or to probe an unclear response.

Q93: ***Snuff or dip tobacco quit attempts lasting longer than 1 day.*** It is important to ensure that R listens to this entire question before answering; otherwise, he or she may answer "Yes" for reasons other than quitting snuff or dip tobacco for a day or longer (e.g., if R was in the hospital for a day or longer).

Methods of Quitting (Snuff or Dip)

Six questions (Q94 to Q99) address methods of quitting snuff or dip tobacco, including nontraditional methods of quitting (Q98). These questions are asked of "current snuff or dip tobacco users" and "former snuff or dip tobacco users." Alternate introductions are provided for the two types of R.

Q94–97: ***Medications used to assist in quitting; "cold turkey" quitting.*** These questions are asked only of "current snuff or dip tobacco users" or "former snuff or dip tobacco users" who quit during the 5 years preceding the interview.

Q98: ***Use of prayer or pledge to assist in quitting.*** This question is asked only of "current snuff or dip tobacco users" or "former snuff or dip tobacco users" who quit during the 5 years preceding the interview.

Q99: ***Use of classes or counseling to assist in quitting.*** This question is asked only of "current snuff or dip tobacco users" who made a quit attempt in the year preceding the interview or of "former snuff or dip tobacco users" who quit during the 5 years preceding the interview.

Readiness to Quit Using Snuff or Dip Tobacco

Three questions (Q100 to Q102) address stages of change for quitting. These questions are asked of "current snuff or dip tobacco users" only.

Q100–102: ***Readiness of R to quit using snuff or dip tobacco.*** These questions are asked only of "current snuff or dip tobacco users."

Physicians' and Health Professionals' Advice to Quit Using Snuff or Dip Tobacco

Eleven questions (Q104 to Q107h) address physicians' and health professionals' advice.

Q103: ***Receipt of health checkup or care in the past 12 months.*** Both "current snuff or dip tobacco users" and "former snuff or dip tobacco users" who quit during the 5 years preceding the interview answer this question.

Q104: ***Health professional's asking whether R uses snuff or dip tobacco.*** This question is asked only of Rs who have seen a health professional in the 12 months preceding the interview ("yes" at Q103).

Q105: ***Health professional's advice not to use snuff or dip tobacco.*** This and subsequent questions in this section are asked only of Rs who answered "yes" at Q103.

Q106a–h: ***Health professional's recommendation to use quit aids.*** This sequence is asked of any R whose health care professional either advised against using snuff or dip tobacco, or asked R whether he or she used snuff or dip tobacco.

2.3.7 Section 7: Secondhand Smoke Exposure

Seven questions (Q107 to Q113) about secondhand smoke establish R's secondhand smoke exposure outside work (Q108 to Q109), workplace secondhand smoke exposure (Q111 to Q113), and attitudes about rules on clean indoor air (Q110).

Q107: ***Number of adults living in R's household.*** This question may prove to be "sensitive" for Rs who live in multifamily households, which sometimes violate maximum-occupancy rules. Interviewers should reassure Rs that their answers are confidential and are used solely for the purpose of research. If R's answer indicates that he or she is counting only his or her own relatives, the interviewer should state that the question is about all adults in the household, whether or not they are related to R.

Q108: ***Number of adult household members who smoke.*** This question is about only tobacco smoking (cigarettes, cigars, or pipes).

Q109: ***Smoking of tobacco inside the home.*** The interviewer should stress the word *inside* to ensure Rs are not including outdoor locations of the home. In cognitive testing, some Rs were including outdoor locations, such as yards.

Q110: ***Rules about smoking inside the home.*** If an R provides an answer that is not one of those listed, the interviewer should reread the categories and ask the R to select from among the responses provided. Responses such as "You can smoke only outside" or "We allow smoking only out in the yard" should be probed, with stress on the word *inside*.

Q111: ***R's working status.*** As part of the general information used to determine whether R should be asked the subsequent questions about smoking in the workplace, this question elicits R's working status. Interviewers should read each response category slowly and give R the opportunity to process each response option; interviewers should read all response options before accepting one as an answer.

Q112: ***R's work location—indoors or not.*** This question is asked to determine whether R should be asked about indoor smoking at work.

Q113: ***Smoking in R's work area.*** No definition is provided for *work area.* It is whatever R defines as his or her work area. Work areas can vary widely. A traveling salesman may consider a car his work area. Other examples of *work area* are cubicle, restaurant dining room, and warehouse.

2.3.8 Section 8: Risk Perception

This section consists of 15 questions (Q114 to Q128) that together cover R's perception of risk from smoking and from secondhand smoke, as well as R's views about prohibiting smoking in specific indoor places. All questions are asked of all Rs.

Q114–128: ***Opinions or knowledge about health risks associated with tobacco use and exposure to secondhand smoke.*** R may feel as though he or she must provide a correct answer to these questions. The interviewer should reassure the R that no "correct" or "incorrect" answers exist for these items, that the researchers are interested in the R's personal opinion.

2.3.9 Section 9: Demographic Items

In this section, six questions (Q129 to Q134) elicit basic demographic information about Rs. They cover R's age, sex, education, household income, sexual identification, and health coverage.

Q129: ***Age.*** Rs occasionally may prefer not to disclose their age. The interviewer should reassure R that responses to the survey are securely protected; then the interviewer should repeat the question.

Q130: ***Sex.*** When certain of the answer, the interviewer may code sex without asking R for it. Whenever uncertain, though, the interviewer must ask. To make asking less awkward, the interviewer may preface the question by saying, "I'm required to ask this question."

Q131: ***Marital status.*** This question determines marital status. Because of the nature of the fishing trade, adult males may be absent for long periods of time. The category *separated* refers only to legal separation, not extended periods of absence.

Q132: ***Children in the home.*** This question refers to the total number of children currently residing in the home, regardless of the relationship of adult householders to the children.

Q133: ***Ethnic heritage of R.*** This question attempts to identify the ethnic heritage of the specific R (not the household). If R is of mixed heritage (has parentage of two different Alaska Native groups) or is only part Alaska Native, select answer code 5 (*multi-ethnic*).

Q134a–b: ***Tribal membership.*** These questions determine whether R is a member (that is, enrolled) in a tribe, a corporation, or a village established under the Indian

Reorganization Act (IRA). If R is, then the interviewer asks the follow-up question, "Which one?" The interviewer should be provided with a list that associates each tribe, corporation, or village name with a number. The appropriate number should be entered in the space provided.

Q135: ***Tribal association.*** Whether or not R is enrolled in a tribe, corporation, or IRA village, the interviewer asks whether R feels a part of any such group. If R does, then the interviewer should enter the code for the tribe, corporation, or IRA village; if R does not, then the interviewer should enter "00" (zero-zero) in the spaces provided.

Q136: ***Native/tribal language use.*** This question and the next seek to determine the language in which R would prefer to communicate. The purpose of these two questions is to help design intervention programs; it is helpful to know what languages could or should be used by program communications and staff. If R says "not much" or "only a little bit" or is otherwise uncertain whether he or she speaks the native (tribal) language, then the interviewer should enter "no" and skip to Q138.

Q137: ***Preferred language.*** This question seeks to determine the language R would be most comfortable communicating in if he or she speaks English and another language. The interviewer should be provided with a list that associates each likely language spoken in the target area with a number 01 to 76, where English is 01. In the space provided, the interviewer should enter the number associated with the preferred language.

Q138: ***Born on island, in village, or in hub.*** This question is to determine whether R was born on the current island (or in the current village or hub if R is not located on an island).

Q139: ***Duration of residence on island (in village or hub).*** This question elicits the length of time R has been a resident of the current island (or village). The interviewer should enter the number of years, rounding to the nearest whole number. If residence has been for less than one year, the interviewer should enter "00"; if it has been for longer than 76 years, the interviewer should enter 76 to signify "76 years or longer."

Q140: ***Highest grade of school completed.*** For this question, the interviewer must elicit the highest grade completed, which will present difficulties when R studied outside the U.S. educational system. Response categories must *not* be read aloud. If R offers as response the level of schooling completed, or degree or title obtained, the interviewer should probe for the total number of years of schooling that level, degree, or title requires in the educational system in which R studied (i.e., how many years were required, starting with the first grade of primary school).

Q141: ***Annual household income.*** With this question, interviewers will find R's annual household income range by reading the list of response categories and waiting for R to stop them at some point. When R stops the interviewer and says something like "Yes, that's it," the interviewer should repeat the category and obtain confirmation. For example, the interviewer can say, "You said $15,001 to $20,000. Is that correct?"

Income can be a "sensitive" topic for many Rs; therefore, the interviewer should be careful to maintain a neutral tone and be prepared to respond to objections. R should be assured that this information is held in strictest confidence.

Interviewers should be clear that R should include all sources of income (e.g., payments from the state or federal government, net income from hunting and fishing).

The income groupings can be scaled down if smaller dollar amounts are more appropriate to the income levels of island or village residents.

Q142: ***Sexual identification.*** This question is about self-identification, not sexual orientation or sexual activities. The interviewer should never paraphrase by asking, for example, whether R is attracted to, or has sex with, men or women. R may be married to someone of the opposite sex yet not self-identify as heterosexual.

If R seems unsure of the meaning of the terms, or reluctant to select, the response is code 4. Code 7 applies only if R says he or she does not know, or is unsure of, which response option best describes him or her but seems to understand the terminology. The interviewer should not interpret or recode answers that are provided in terms completely different from the allowable response categories. For example, in cognitive testing, responses included "I'm a man, a complete man." In such cases, the interviewer should reread the answer categories and ask R to select from the listed options.

Q143: ***Health insurance coverage.*** The qualifying sentence after the question is intended to exclude free or reduced-cost clinics for low-income Rs. The question pertains only to private or government-sponsored health coverage plans.

2.3.10 Section 10: User-Selected Items

While the AN ATS features a set of core questions, all of which should be administered, the model provides for researchers' addition of user-selected items uniquely relevant to the local community in which the survey will be conducted. Users of the AN ATS are invited to add questions to the end of the AN ATS to gain information about topics of local concern. Other AN ATS users have added questions on topics such as diabetes, exposure to smoke when in a vehicle (e.g., driving with other workers to a construction site), opinions about smoking in specific buildings in the community, and parental intervention in children's smoking.

Selection of additional questions begins with the identification of topics of interest as determined by the study's objectives. Adequate time should be built into the survey schedule for discussions among the investigators, analysts, program administrators, and health professionals to decide the most important topics of local concern that are not already addressed in earlier sections of the questionnaire.

After the topics of interest have been honed, the next step is finding tested, validated questions on the topic. Writing original questions is discouraged, especially because a large selection of tobacco-use and health-related questions already exists. Survey questions may be taken from databases such as the Question Inventory on Tobacco (QIT). This Web-based tool was developed by the Centers for Disease Control and Prevention's Office on Smoking and Health and houses tobacco-related questions. These questions may require cognitive testing for the feasibility of use with the Alaska Native population.

Well-regarded, validated survey questionnaires that offer questions on a wide range of topics include the following:

- ***The Behavioral Risk Factor Surveillance System (BRFSS).*** BRFSS is the world's largest, ongoing telephone health survey system, tracking health conditions and risk behaviors in the United States; data are collected monthly in all 50 states, including Alaska (Centers for Disease Control and Prevention, 2009).

- ***The National Health and Nutrition Examination Survey (NHANES).*** NHANES is a program of studies designed to assess the health and nutritional status of adults and children in the United States. Smoking, alcohol consumption, sexual practices, drug use, physical fitness and activity, weight, and dietary intake are studied (Centers for Disease Control and Prevention, National Center for Health Statistics, 2008).

- ***The National Health Interview Survey (NHIS).*** NHIS, conducted by the National Center for Health Statistics, monitors a broad range of health topics by means of household interviews (Centers for Disease Control and Prevention, National Centers for Health Statistics, 2008).

The final selection of additional questions should be added to the end of the questionnaire, in the section titled "User-selected Items." Placing questions in other modules may upset the underlying logic of the interview and disrupt the skip patterns. Preservation of the skip patterns is essential to directing Rs to the right questions.

User-selected items should be limited in number so that the total length of administration does not greatly exceed 30 minutes. As a rule, the participant will complete four to six questions per minute. More than a few minutes of additional questions may result in a reduced response rate. Users are cautioned against deleting any core questions in an effort to reduce the length of the questionnaire. Dropping questions could compromise the analyses that are possible and could disrupt the skip patterns.

In addition to being limited in number, the additional items should be on similar, health-related topics: Surveys that cover too wide an array of topics can also lead to nonresponse.

Additional questions and any other modifications made to the AN ATS, especially formatting changes, should take into account the ease with which the questionnaire can be completed by the interviewer and the method used for key-entering responses.

2.4 Advance Letters

Introductory letters may be mailed to households in advance of the interviewer's visit. Many survey researchers have found that advance letters improve cooperation and reduce the number of contacts required to complete the survey (Dillman, 2000). An advance letter should describe the survey and explain why it is important.

The essential components of an advance letter are

- an explanation of the survey,

- identification of the sponsoring organization,

- the purpose for collecting the data, and

- an explanation of how the data will be used.

A sample advance letter has been provided (Appendix A). It should be modified to reflect the specific circumstances of a survey. For example, the letter may be modified to include a message about the voluntary nature of survey participation, the ability of the R to skip questions he or she does not want to answer, and an assurance of the security of the data. Any compensation for R's time (monetary or otherwise) should be mentioned in the letter. Providing the name of the sponsoring agency or data collection organization often fosters the R's confidence in the study.

If the sample members for an in-person survey live very near each other, it may be easiest for interviewers to simply distribute advance letters under doors before they start ringing any doorbells. If the names and addresses of survey members are known, then personalized letters can be sent via regular mail. If the list contains addresses but no names, the letter should be addressed to the household without naming any specific person. Because this method is not as effective as an individually addressed letter, it is important to ensure that the outside of the envelope looks like an important communication, one not easily confused with "junk mail."

Whatever method is used to deliver it, the advance letter is typically dispatched so that it arrives about 2 weeks before the interviewer first contacts the household. If mailed too early, it may be forgotten by the time the household is contacted for the interview. Mailed too close to the contact date, it may not yet have been received or read. Interviewers should also carry a copy of the advance letter with them to provide to participants who request one.

2.5 Household Screener

The AN ATS Household Screener (Appendix B) contains a brief introduction to the AN ATS and poses several questions designed to accomplish the following:

- verify that the interviewer is at the correct household,

- establish the eligibility of the household to participate (one or more household members must be an Alaska Native),

- select a household member at random to be interviewed from among all eligible persons in the household, and

- prompt the interviewer to obtain informed consent from the R before the interview begins.

In addition, the AN ATS Household Screener introduces the interviewer to the R. The R learns that the survey has been approved by the village or corporation board. The script reinforces, as well, the importance of the R's help in fulfilling the aims of the study.

2.6 Informed Consent

A signed informed consent statement is required from every R to ensure that all Rs are aware of their rights as participants and that when they agree to participate they do so with a clear understanding of what will be involved. The informed consent provides detailed information about what Rs are being asked to do, why the research is necessary and important, what participation actually entails, how Rs' privacy and security will be protected, and the risks or benefits that may result from participating. The consent statement should be written at an easy reading level. Rs are provided the name and contact information for someone who can answer questions about their rights as participants in a survey.

A sample of an informed consent form is provided (Appendix C). It should be customized to suit each survey's particular circumstances. The body sanctioning the specific survey, usually an institutional review board (IRB), should review and approve the customized informed consent to ensure that it is thorough and accurate (for more information about the roles of an IRB, see Section 3.4). The informed consent protects the survey organization and survey sponsor from any future claims that a participant was unaware of what participation would entail or its risks.

The informed consent statement is read by (or to) the R, who must sign it before the interview can begin. If the R does not want to give formal consent to participate, the interviewer must not begin the interview. Typically, the R will need to sign the informed consent form if the R agrees to participate. The study's IRB will decide whether a signed consent form must be obtained, or whether verbal consent is sufficient.

Low-literacy populations may have problems reading and interpreting the written consent form. To make the situation less awkward, the interviewer may say, "I'm going to read this to you, unless you prefer to read it yourself." In addition, interviewers must be able to explain terms in the consent and respond to any questions the R might have. Interviewers should pay attention to verbal and nonverbal indications that the R may be having difficulty understanding what he or she is reading or hearing. In these cases, the interviewer should take extra time to explain the terms of the consent.

2.7 "Sorry I Missed You" Card

Whenever the interviewer arrives at a participant's home and finds that the residents are away, the interviewer leaves a "Sorry I Missed You" card to inform the participant that the interviewer visited to conduct the interview. The card should provide a telephone number for the participant to call to reschedule the interview (Appendix E).

2.8 Receipt

For interview participation, a token of appreciation in the form of check or a gift card may be offered to study participants. To help track incentive awards paid to Rs, a sample receipt card is provided (Appendix F).

3.   SURVEY PLANNING AND BUDGETING

Good planning is essential to the successful completion of a survey. Whether the user's organization is planning to perform the survey independently, or planning to hire a contracting company, knowing what must be accomplished is important. This chapter covers some of the more important matters the survey team should consider when planning a survey.

3.1   Instrumentation

Perhaps the most important feature of the survey is the questionnaire. It is strongly recommended that the Alaska Native Adult Tobacco Survey (AN ATS) be used in its entirety. The AN ATS was carefully designed and tested to elicit population-based, community-specific information on the prevalence of commercial tobacco use and commercial tobacco-use behaviors, knowledge, attitudes, and beliefs among Alaska Natives. It embodies both accepted scientific practice and interviewing strategies culturally specific to Alaska Natives; it is the foundation on which to build a comprehensive tobacco-use survey research program.

The AN ATS has some limitations that are important to remember. The AN ATS covers tobacco-related topics and was designed as a paper questionnaire to be administered in person to Alaska Natives. The AN ATS may not be relevant, culturally appropriate, or applicable to other population groups or serve other informational objectives. The AN ATS has not been tested for administration in other modes, such as telephone or self-administered interviewing.

3.2   Survey Protocol Checklists

Sound survey research design requires protocols for key survey activities. Early development of protocols and procedures provides the framework for survey success. Observance of these protocols fosters consistent, rigorous performance of survey operations, which enforces the scientific validity of the research findings. Formal, written survey protocols are a helpful reference for team members and are required for institutional review board (IRB) approval.

Checklists are provided here to aid researchers in organizing survey protocols and identifying survey design issues. Not every item is applicable to every survey. Many of the listed items are discussed in greater detail elsewhere in this guidance document.

3.2.1 Project Overview Checklist

- Formulate a title.

- Draft a project summary.

- Determine name, location, and contact information for investigators, collaborators, and funding sources.

- Determine name of the IRB or governing body responsible for protecting participants' rights.

3.2.2 Introduction Checklist

- Define the current state of knowledge about survey topics (i.e., what is known about tobacco use in the survey target area).

- Formulate informational objectives (i.e., specify the knowledge sought).

- Formulate hypotheses or questions (not necessarily formal hypotheses, but at least the kinds of results that would be meaningful or would lead to specified actions).

- Determine intended and potential uses of survey findings.

- Describe the organization to conduct the survey (general approach to project management, staffing, facilities, and additional resources such as subcontractors, university resources, and the like).

3.2.3 Survey Design Checklist

- Describe the survey design and show how it supports the informational objectives, answers the research questions, and tests any hypotheses formulated.

- Describe the involvement and contributions of the survey team and the efforts to involve stakeholders and community members.

- Discuss how information will improve the effectiveness of health programs in the survey target area and among Alaska Natives.

- Draft a study timeline.

- Delineate steps to obtain a review of the survey protocols from an IRB or other governing body.

3.2.4 Study Population Checklist

- Describe the survey population and survey target area.

- Identify the unit of observation in the survey.

- Articulate criteria for participant eligibility.

- Provide justification for any exclusion of a subsegment of the population.

- Describe the sampling plan, including sample size, expected response rate, and measure of statistical power. Include any limitations to the sample (i.e., sample frame may exclude persons not on the community list) and the measures taken to compensate for these limitations (e.g., comparison of the community list with other lists to discover names missing from the community list).

- Describe how survey participants will be enlisted.

3.2.5 *Instrumentation Checklist*

- Identify key variables and constructs (e.g., definition of a *smoker*).

- Attach survey materials, including the AN ATS, any site-specific questions added to the AN ATS, and all survey forms.

- Describe plans for interviewer training; attach a training manual.

- Describe plans for training all persons involved in the survey in confidentiality procedures; attach training materials.

3.2.6 *Data Collection, Tabulation, and Analysis Checklist*

- Describe plans for collecting data from participants.

- Describe plans for analysis of the survey data, including planned tables and figures.

- Identify the software packages to be used to (1) organize and maintain administrative records, (2) create electronic files of survey data, and (3) analyze the data.

- Describe procedures for (1) preparing data for data entry, (2) performing data entry (i.e., batching questionnaires), (3) editing keyed data for accuracy and consistency, and (4) reporting on problems found in data (e.g., a question consistently answered erroneously).

- Describe measures to ensure the confidentiality of the survey responses, the privacy of respondent information, and the physical security of completed questionnaires and electronic records.

- Discuss biases possibly produced in findings during data collection, data-set building, or analyses.

- Discuss any other possible limitations to the survey findings, their representativeness, or their generalizability.

3.2.7 *Unexpected or Adverse Events Checklist*

- Describe how unexpected events (e.g., severe weather) may affect the ability to conduct the survey; determine the response to such challenges (e.g., consultation with team members and revision of survey schedule).

- Describe how adverse events will be managed and documented; note whether adverse events must be reported to the IRB or other governing body.

- Describe resources for providing emergency care to survey staff, interviewers, or participants if such care is needed during survey operations.

3.2.8 Dissemination Checklist

- Describe plans for sharing survey results with (1) participants, (2) community members, (3) other stakeholders, (4) team members, and (5) other interested researchers (i.e., at conference presentations).

- Describe any plans to disseminate actual survey data files outside the survey research team, with particular attention to how the data will be kept confidential and how participants' privacy will be ensured.

3.3 Survey Implementation: Community Engagement

The first step in implementing the AN ATS is to engage stakeholders and secure the buy-in of tribal leaders and community members. One of the best ways to do so is to acknowledge and respect that the participating tribe is a sovereign nation.

Another key to buy-in is to ensure that tribal leaders have a clear understanding of the survey project; survey staff members must be prepared to make presentations throughout the tribal community. These presentations should explain the cultural appropriateness of the AN ATS, as well as its background, purpose, and procedures. Presentations to tribal councils and communities also can demonstrate how the community will participate in and benefit from the survey. Presenters should remind survey participants that the survey is owned by the tribal community, so the tribal community will decide how its AN ATS findings are used.

Survey staff members are encouraged to make presentations at community meetings, to communicate through tribal and clinic newsletters, and to work with community gatekeepers to share information about the survey project. (For a sample letter requesting permission to engage the tribal community, see Appendix A.)

3.4 Institutional Review Board Approval

Before the AN ATS is implemented, it may be necessary to submit the survey protocol to an IRB, or other governing body, for review and approval. In the United States, IRB review and approval is required for all research that receives funding, directly or indirectly, from the U.S. Department of Health and Human Services.

The primary role of the IRB is to protect the rights of research participants. It does so by confirming that the survey protocol respects the rights of individuals to refuse to participate, does not harm the participant in any way, and does not unfairly burden any participant. The criteria used by an IRB to evaluate a research study include the following:

- The protocol must be scientifically sound and worthwhile.

- Risks must be minimized to the extent possible.

- Subjects must be selected equitably.

- Informed consent must be obtained.

- Privacy and confidentiality must be protected.

- The study must be adequately monitored.

IRB review and approval serve two additional objectives. IRB approval of protocols helps protect the sponsoring agency (or company contracted to conduct the survey) if a participant feels his or her rights were violated. Furthermore, a statement of protocols is imperative for defining the responsibilities of the organization conducting the survey.

The AN ATS is a survey that involves human subjects; therefore, after a tribe has granted permission for the survey, the organization administering the survey must obtain IRB approval, as well. Some tribes or corporations may already have an IRB, so the project coordinator should work with tribal or corporation leadership to determine the proper steps to take to receive IRB approval from the tribe. If a tribe or corporation has no IRB, the project coordinator should seek approval from the Indian Health Services, because of its extensive knowledge, skills, and abilities in working with tribes in the United States (the Indian Health Services IRB can contacted by e-mail at irb@ihs.org).

Either way, the project coordinator must work with the tribal organization or corporation to determine which organization is available to provide this approval. The IRB approval process should begin early, preferably immediately after a tribe gives permission to conduct the survey, because this process can take a long time.

While the project director is responsible for obtaining IRB approval, the survey manager is typically responsible for preparing materials submitted to the IRB. The director and manager should consult the IRB chairperson to learn what materials the IRB requires.

Research participants are typically provided telephone numbers (local or toll-free) for both the project manager (for questions about the study) and the IRB or governing body (for questions about participants' rights). The IRB must maintain records of all communications with research subjects (U.S. Department of Health and Human Services, 2008).

3.5 Data Ownership and Data Sharing

Many tribes have policies and procedures in place to protect data and information generated by research, surveys, and other types of data collection, especially data collection conducted by external organizations. These policies and procedures may be overseen by entities—such as tribal and regional IRB or research and information subcommittees—created under the doctrine of sovereignty. It is recommended that AN ATS project staff inquire about such policies and procedures and work with the respective organizations to adhere to them.

Data-sharing agreements are an important part of any data collection, but, because of tribal sovereignty and the need to prevent the misuse of collected data, these agreements are even more significant for studies among Alaska Native populations. AN ATS project staff should work with tribal leaders, tribal organizations, and community members to determine the content of any data-sharing agreements, as well as the ways to secure the data. This approach may entail working with the tribe to develop safeguards to protect the data.

Although tribal community members should staff the survey project, the organization administering the survey may need to engage researchers, analysts, and staff from outside the tribal community to help with survey implementation. Data-sharing agreements ensure that all parties understand privacy issues, data ownership, and corresponding concerns, such as publication rights and dissemination through presentations.

3.6 Survey Location

The AN ATS was developed for in-person interviewing, which means that interviewers conduct the survey personally rather than by telephone or mail; therefore, the survey protocols must establish where the surveys can be conducted. Most in-person surveys are conducted in the respondent's home. When the respondent's home is used, the protocols must address issues of safety and privacy for both the interviewer and the respondent. Arrangements may be made for conducting interviews in alternative locations more convenient for the respondent. Any alternative location must be one providing adequate privacy, such as a private office in a clinic or administration building. Public places, such as restaurants, may not provide adequate privacy.

3.7 Survey Staffing

Conducting a survey is a multifaceted process requiring much work by many people. Delineated here is a possible staffing pattern. The precise job positions are relatively unimportant, however; what matters most is that someone be assigned to each responsibility described.

3.7.1 Principal Investigator

Many survey projects are led by a *principal investigator* (PI). A PI is not essential, though. Survey efforts organize themselves in different ways, depending on the structure of the team and the availability of staff. Often, decisions are reached through a group consensus process considering the needs of the survey sponsors, program administrators, and other stakeholders. Either way, one set of responsibilities often rests with the PI: applying for and obtaining IRB approvals, informing the IRB of any protocol changes or revisions, and informing the IRB of any reportable adverse events. These responsibilities must be covered in the survey staffing plan.

PIs are also often made responsible for the initial analysis of survey findings. Because survey results are often limited to descriptive presentations, an experienced analyst with a good analysis plan may suffice, depending on available resources.

3.7.2 Project Coordinator

The staff member most central to a survey team is the *project coordinator* (PC). In some circumstances, the PI and PC roles are combined into one job. Alternatively, a PC's responsibilities may be effectively distributed among several persons, so long as all PC duties are assigned to specific staff and fulfilled. These responsibilities are as follows:

- to prepare survey protocols;

- to assist in preparing questions for the User-selected Items module and ensuring that they are properly added to the survey questionnaire;

- to fulfill managerial and administrative roles on the survey, including management of survey staff, recruitment and management of interviewers, and monitoring of staff performance;

- to participate in meetings, training programs, and workshops with survey team partners;

- to coordinate with local stakeholders, particularly if the group will be assisting in the protocol (e.g., helping to select additional questions, providing a location for interviews to be conducted);

- to train and supervise staff on key activities, such as sampling, interviewing, and using software;

- to train staff for cultural competency in working with local populations;

- to ensure that confidentiality and data management procedures are properly performed;

- to account for the staff's financial expenditures, including the funds for incentives;

- to oversee implementation of project procedures and data collection procedures; and

- to help disseminate findings both through local channels and by other means.

The PC should be someone with considerable knowledge of the survey target community, sound understanding of health-related research issues, notable leadership skills, survey experience, and careful attention to detail. Also helpful in a PC is familiarity with the computer applications to be used in survey processes such as word processing, spreadsheets, file management, data entry, and data analysis. Finally, studies benefit from having a PC known and respected in the local community, because the PC will regularly interface with community members and other stakeholders.

3.7.3 Field Supervisor

Depending on the size of the survey, one or more persons should be designated *field supervisor* (FS). Because the FS must be well organized and able to work well with an entire staff of interviewers, it is recommended that the FS come to the position with survey experience and experience in managing field staff. The roles and responsibilities of a field supervisor are as follows:

- to schedule interviewers' time and decide which interviewers will go to which households;

- to provide assistance to interviewers to work through any problems encountered in the field;

- to distribute and track incentives if they are to be provided to participants;

- to report regularly on survey progress, including number of completed interviews to date, completion rates for each interviewer, and expense reports;

- to ensure that all interviewers carefully follow protocols and procedures;

- to ensure the confidentiality and security of completed questionnaires, as well as electronic files and all other survey materials;

- to conduct quality control checks, which may include randomly accompanying interviewers on visits to households, reviewing interviewers' work for accuracy, and calling to confirm that an interviewer actually conducted the interview whose responses were submitted; and

- to provide for interviewer retraining as needed and to recruit and train new interviewers if current staff must be replaced.

3.7.4 Interviewers

Interviewers should be highly motivated and able and willing to work outside the office and outside normal business hours, which may include evening and weekend hours. Interviewers should be knowledgeable and culturally competent in terms of the local community and Alaska Natives residing in it. To the extent possible, interviewers should be representative of the racial and ethnic minority populations in the community. If the target community is small, some protocol should be in place so that interviewers do not interview people they know personally. Interviewers must be able to address participants' concerns and properly conduct the interview, thereby assuring the collection of high-quality, complete data.

3.8   Budgeting

Provided here is a budget template for an in-person household survey with paper questionnaires. It will remind the user what kind of staff members may be required and expenses that may be incurred. Not all items listed will be relevant to every project; types of expenses may vary.

3.8.1 Survey Administration and Operations Staff (Labor Costs)

- principal investigator
- project coordinator
- training instructors
- field supervisors
- interviewers
- data entry staff
- data analyst/programmer
- report writer
- graphics / word processing support

3.8.2 Survey Planning Costs

- travel and expenses for team members to attend group meetings
- long-distance charges for teleconferences
- facility charges for meetings
- rental charges for audiovisual equipment
- food and miscellaneous expenses related to meetings
- copies of materials for meetings, binders, and the like
- delivery or mailing costs

3.8.3 Training Costs

- copies of training manual and other training materials
- rental charges for training rooms
- rental charges for audiovisual equipment
- food and miscellaneous expenses related to training
- travel of trainers to and from training site
- travel of interviewers to and from training site
- lodging and per diem costs

- honorarium or wages for trainers and interviewers

- travel and expenses for others who plan to attend training

- delivery or mailing costs

3.8.4 Data Collection Costs

- advance letter addressing, printing, stuffing, and mailing

- travel and expenses for field interviewers to recruit households and conduct surveys

- travel and expenses for fss to monitor staff in field

- copies of survey materials, including questionnaires, cards, and the like.

- supplies for the field (photo ids, locked bags or other materials for storing confidential records, maps, records of calls, "Sorry I Missed You" cards, business cards, timesheets, and the like)

- cell phones for interviewers

- incentive payments for participants

- long-distance charges

- locking storage cabinets (to secure questionnaires)

- delivery or mailing costs

- long-term storage for questionnaires and data files

3.8.5 Dissemination Costs

- Graphics for reports

- Copies of reports and other materials

- Printing and binding

- Hosting of meetings with stakeholders to deliver or discuss findings

- Travel and expenses for meeting attendees

- Delivery or mailing costs

3.9 Work Plan and Schedule

Provided here is an example of a detailed work plan with approximate "days to complete" (Table 3-1). Many of the listed activities can be conducted concurrently, depending on the availability of staff. Local circumstances will likewise affect the time required to perform tasks. When building a schedule, the user should be sure to include time for both performing tasks and having materials reviewed by all relevant decision makers.

Table 3-1. Sample Task List / Work Plan

Task/Subtask	Work Days
Complete sampling design and obtain lists	
Decide on sampling plan	30
Develop sampling design	8
Obtain person list or household list	60
Implement sampling design	10
Develop data collection materials	
Complete Interviewer training manual	40
Complete field supervisor manual	40
Complete survey brochure	20
Compile news articles about the study	20
Complete frequently asked questions	20
Complete receipt forms	20
Complete door hanger that says "Sorry I Missed You"	20
Complete advance letter	20
Complete field interviewer authorization letter	20
Complete field interviewer confidentiality pledge	20
Complete field interviewer transmittal sheet	20
Complete noninterview report form	20
Complete paper screening form	20
Complete consent forms	20
Complete show cards	20
Obtain institutional review board (IRB) approvals	
Develop and submit IRB protocol	30
Obtain IRB approval[a]	60
Purchase equipment and supplies	
Finalize equipment selection	1
Order and purchase shoulder/rolling bags	30
Print data collection materials[b]	20
Assemble case folders	5
Quality control case folders	2
Staffing	
Develop field supervisor recruitment and hiring materials	30
Screen and interview field supervisory staff	30
Hire field supervisory staff	30
Develop field interviewer recruitment and hiring materials	30
Screen and interview field interviewers	30
Hire field interviewers	30

(continued)

Table 3-1.   Sample Task List / Work Plan (continued)

Task/Subtask	Work Days
Prepare for and conduct training	
Arrange logistics for trainings	20
Identify and reserve training and hotel facilities	15
Make travel arrangements	15
Develop training agendas	20
Develop supervisor and interviewer training materials	20
Hold supervisors' training session	5
Print interviewer training agenda and materials	5
Mail home study packets	1
Hold field interviewers' training	10
Hold attrition training	10
Print and send advance letters	
Prepare name and address information	1/2
Print, stuff, and mail	2
Allow mailing delivery time	7
Collect data	180
Conduct verifications[c]	30
Perform quality control[d]	30
Receive and process data	
Produce deliverables	180
Wrap up; prepare final data file	30

[a] The number of days to complete depends on how often the IRB convenes.

[b] The number of days to complete depends on the printer.

[c] Distributed throughout data collection.

[d] Distributed throughout data collection.

A Gantt chart, illustrated next, is a particularly effective way to display multiple, overlapping tasks and to graphically indicate which tasks depend on earlier tasks before they can be begun (Figure 3-1).

jure 3-1. Sample Gantt Chart

Tasks	Months After Project Award																			
	1	2	3	4	5	6	7	8	9	10	11	12	13	14	15	16	17	18	19	20
Complete sampling design and obtain lists	▆	▆	▆	▆	▆															
Develop data collection materials	▆																			
Obtain IRB approvals		▆	▆	▆	▆															
Develop and submit IRB protocol		▆																		
Obtain IRB approval			▆	▆	▆															
Print data collection materials						▆														
Purchase equipment and supplies						▆														
Staffing					▆	▆	▆	▆												
Prepare for and conduct training								▆	▆											
Print and send advance letters									▆											
Collect data										▆	▆	▆	▆	▆	▆	▆	▆			
Conduct verifications											▆	▆	▆	▆	▆	▆	▆			
Quality control											▆	▆	▆	▆	▆	▆	▆			
Receive and process data											▆	▆	▆	▆	▆	▆	▆			
Wrap up; prepare final data file																		▆	▆	

3.1□ □□pe□ting the □ne□pe□te□

Every survey will present its own unexpected challenges, so flexibility and readiness to address changing circumstances are important. Availability of senior staff, weather contingencies, and interviewer safety are three areas that benefit from planning ahead.

3.10.1 Availability of Senior Project Staff

Working well with people requires considerable flexibility and a willingness to accommodate special circumstances. Because they are in the field, interviewers are the first to try to address problems that arise. Interviewers should consult with their supervisors, however, when confronted with difficult or novel situations. In turn, supervisors should help solve more difficult problems. Moreover, even when supervisors feel they can resolve a situation, they should consult with the PC to be sure the solution abides by the survey protocols as approved by the IRB.

Because many problems require immediate solutions, interviewers must to be able to contact supervisors, and supervisors must be able to contact coordinators so an acceptable decision can be made without delay. Because many surveys will be conducted after normal business hours, supervisors and coordinators must be accessible on nights and weekends.

3.10.2 Scheduling and the Weather

Conducting the AN ATS may be challenged by severe weather because interviewers must be outdoors, going door-to-door. The schedule for fishing and crop seasons can also limit interviewers' access to respondents. Only a narrow window of time may exist for reaching respondents. The schedule for the survey field effort must accommodate such limitations.

3.10.3 Interviewer Safety

The safety of the interviewing staff must be paramount among concerns. Two measures used successfully on other surveys are (1) the "buddy system," so no interviewer enters a respondent's home alone, and (2) the check-in system, whereby the interviewer contacts his or her supervisor just before entering a home and immediately after leaving.

Interviewers should make every effort to interview all sampled persons. If a respondent is hostile or says or does anything that makes an interviewer fear for his or her own safety, the interviewer should leave the respondent's home immediately and report the encounter to his or her supervisor.

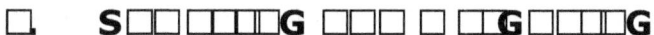

For the Alaska Native Adult Tobacco Survey (AN ATS) to provide meaningful information that can be used to guide and evaluate intervention programs, the findings must represent the target population. This chapter provides basic information about scientifically sound sampling methods appropriate for Alaska Native populations. It is recommended that a sampling statistician be consulted.

The target population for the AN ATS is all civilian, noninstitutionalized Alaska Native residents aged 18 years or older. The total population of Alaska as of the 2000 U.S. Census was 626,932. Approximately 15.6% of the population in Alaska was American Indian or Alaska Native. The composition of the population for other race/ethnicity groups was as follows:

- 69.4% white

- 3.5% black

- 4.0% Asian

- 0.5% Native Hawaiian or other Pacific Islander

- 1.6% "other" single-race households[1]

The balance of the population in Alaska was 5.4% and consisted of persons residing in a household with two or more races represented.

Typically, population-based probability samples are based on one of two kinds of lists: one of all target community members (list sample), or one of all target community households (area sample). Because Alaska Natives represent only 15.6% of the Alaskan population and are sparsely located throughout the state, for the AN ATS a cost-effective method of drawing the sample is by individual member rather than area household. An appropriate list of members may be available from tribal leaders or other sources.

When the survey sample is based on lists of individual members rather than on households, the "long" version of the AN ATS should be used because it assumes possession of the respondents' names. Conversely, when households are sampled and eventual participants' names are therefore unknown, the "short" version of the AN ATS should be used, preceded by use of the In-Person Screener for Selection of Eligible Household Respondent. The In-Person Screener steps the interviewer through selection of a household resident to

---

[1]This chapter adopts the survey definitions used in the 2000 U.S. Census: A *dwelling unit* (HU) is a house, an apartment, a mobile home or trailer, a group of rooms, or a single room occupied as separate living quarters or, if vacant, intended for occupancy as separate living quarters. A *household* includes all persons who occupy a HU as their usual place of residence. A *householder* is the person, or one of the persons, in whose name the home is owned, being bought, or rented.

interview; it also provides the sampling statistician with the information required to assign a probability of selection to that respondent.

4.1 Sampling Individual Persons From a Community List

If the lists of persons are available, the first task is to ascertain their completeness. All ineligible members, such as persons younger than 18 years of age, should be removed from the lists. Conversely, efforts should be made to assess whether all Alaska Native residents of the target area have been included. This task may involve checking multiple lists and cross-referencing them to produce a single complete list.

Once the list is complete, a systematic sampling method should be used.

Systematic sampling is necessary to produce a proportionate sample. Proportionate sampling will yield a self-weighting sample and the members will generally appear in the sample at the same rate as that at which they appear in the population.

4.2 Area Sampling

Often a list of community members does not exist and cannot be easily built. In these circumstances, multistage area sampling offers a form of probability sampling in which recognized geopolitical area units are selected as part of the process of selecting the final survey sample (see Kish, 1995). Area sampling is commonly used to select HUs in In-Person sample surveys. Area samples are most useful when the target area of the survey can be subdivided into a reasonably large number of geopolitical subunits with well-defined boundaries and when population counts, maps, and other statistical data are readily available.

4.2.1 Sample Design

If a complete list of community members cannot be found or developed, a stratified two-stage cluster sample of HUs is recommended. Individual block groups (BGs) should be designated as primary sampling units (PSUs) for random selection in the first stage.[2] Within each selected PSU, a separate simple random sample of HUs should be chosen as secondary sampling units (SSUs). When persons in each sample HU are selected, the resulting set of selected persons is considered a stratified three-stage cluster sample of persons.

---

[2]BGs are clusters of Census blocks. Across the United States, a BG contains about 600 to 3,000 persons, with an average size of 1,500 persons and about 200 to 1,200 households. For a more detailed definition, see the U.S. Census glossary (U.S. Census Bureau, n.d.). In Alaska each BG contains about 139 to 7,381 persons, with a mean of 1,176 persons. Each Alaskan BG has about 64 to 1,917 households, with a mean of 490 household. Of these households, about 1 to 442 households have a member who is an Alaska Native, with a mean of 50.

Sa□□ing □ra□e□

One of the goals of a scientifically sound survey is to ensure that findings from the survey can be generalized to the target population from which the sample was drawn. To accomplish this goal, the sample selected should be representative of the target population, and each sampling unit should have a known nonzero probability of selection. Because a sampling frame is the list, or lists, from which a sample is selected, the construction of representative sampling frames is important in the implementation of the AN ATS.

Sele□ti□n □□Pri□ary Sa□□ing □nit□

Area household sampling begins with a list of PSUs. The PSU sampling frame should be the list of all BGs in the specific target area as given in the most recent decennial Census. For example, a statewide study would comprise all 533 BGs in Alaska. A smaller area, such as a town or community, would include only those BGs captured within the boundary of the town or community.

The SSU sampling frame for each sample PSU is the best possible listing of all households in the PSU. A simple random sample is applied to each PSU household listing; then selected households are contacted and screened for Alaska Natives. The sampling frame for the third-stage selection should be the list of all eligible Alaska Native adults within selected SSUs. This frame of household members derives from a roster of members from sample households.

4.2.2 Primary Sampling Unit Construction and Selection

PSU stratification may be used for any of the following reasons:

- To improve the precision of overall estimates of the target population.[3]

- To ensure geographic representation of the target population in the sample.[4]

- To oversample key population subgroups.

The PSU frame construction should include several important variables for each BG: total population, total households, and totals for the population and households where one or more householders are Alaska Native.

Once the final set of stratification variables is determined, a cross-classification of these variables defines a set of strata for PSU selection. To choose PSU samples in each stratum independently, a stratum identifier, □ is affixed to each member of the final PSU frame.

---

[3]Precision improves in this way to the extent that the variables used for stratification are statistically correlated with the major outcome variables of the study. Smoking is thought to be correlated with gender, socioeconomic level, and population density; therefore, the block groups may be stratified by one or more of these characteristics to increase the precision of the estimates.
[4]Boroughs and Census areas can be used for this purpose.

Because BGs vary widely in size, they should be chosen with probabilities proportional to the 2000 population size of Alaska Natives.

The experience gained from previously completed surveys can help guide the decision about the number of PSUs for allocation. A good rule to follow is as follows: the greater the number of sample PSUs one can afford, the better the statistical results will be from the sample. A minimum of 100 sample PSUs is recommended if the emphasis of analysis is on statewide estimates. On the other hand, if specific interest is in producing sound substate Alaska estimates (e.g., by each of several groupings of boroughs or Census areas), a minimum of 50 PSUs should be selected in each such substate area.

Oversampling of areas containing a higher density of Alaska Natives may be considered for a statewide survey or survey covering a large portion of the state. Oversampling is used in large surveys to increase the percentage of sample households that contain members of the targeted population. This technique can, however, result in some losses in the precision of survey estimates. The gains in precision arising from interviewing a larger number of Alaska Natives must be balanced, therefore, against the overall estimation precision loss due to oversampling (Kalsbeek, 2003). Oversampling will make the household screening more efficient in that a larger percentage of households screened for race/ethnicity will be Alaska Native than would be the case if all households were sampled proportionately. Consequently, the sample size of Alaska Natives will be greater for fixed screening costs and, therefore, contribute to improvements in the precision of survey estimates. On the other hand, unequal probabilities of selection can reduce the precision of survey estimates, such as overall state estimates.

Stratification by other block-level characteristics available from the 2000 Census may also improve the precision of estimates for Alaska Natives, provided such characteristics are correlated with smoking behavior measures of interest for Alaska Native populations. Sex, socioeconomic level of the area, population density, and other known correlates of smoking behavior may be considered for this purpose.

Deciding whether oversampling or stratification is right for a specific survey requires careful consideration of both statistical and practical implications. For example, identifying and oversampling high-density areas for a survey covering a small area of the state or areas where Alaska Natives are fairly evenly distributed will improve precision very little. It is recommended that a sampling statistician, a survey methodologist, or both consider the pros and cons of different sampling plans before a final decision is made (Cochran, 1977).

4.2.3 Secondary Sampling Unit Construction and Selection

The objectives of second-stage sampling are to

- Provide an accurate enumeration of HUs currently located in the target area and

- Describe the sampling procedures for randomly selecting HUs.

Described here are ways to make complete lists and to sample from these lists.

Se□□ndary Sa□□ing □nit □ra□e □□n□tru□ti□n

The frame for choosing dwellings may be constructed in several ways. The traditional HU listing approach has been to have trained field staff walk past every dwelling unit (DU) in the target area and record the address (or a description that could be used to locate the DU later; Kish, 1995, sec. 9.6). Field staff begin at the place on the block shown by the X in the upper-right (i.e., northeast) corner of a sketch sheet map of the BG to be listed. From this starting point HUs are enumerated as they are encountered on the right as the fieldworker proceeds generally in a clockwise direction around the block, or blocks. Listed HUs are limited to those located inside the boundaries of the BG. Identified HUs are marked on the sketch sheet, and their addresses or descriptions are listed in the same order on a separate sheet. Special attention must be paid to some special situations, such as the order for listing unnumbered dwellings within one building, listing vacant dwellings and dwellings under construction, and BGs containing no dwellings. The list of all HUs becomes the frame for sample selection in the second stage.

Although this approach produces a useful frame, it is relatively expensive to implement because specially trained fieldworkers must travel to the selected BGs to do the listing. A possibly more efficient, less expensive alternative to using HU listings alone is to use postal mailing lists and property tax parcel listings to generate the primary list for enumerating the HU sample. A particularly attractive approach produces a full enumeration by using a combination of tax parcel records and USPS residential mailing address data (where available and affordable) for those HUs thought to exist within the boundaries of the sample BGs. Initial listings of HUs may be obtained from a reputable vendor (e.g., MSG-Genesys) for those sample PSUs (BGs) where USPS postal carrier lists of addresses are reasonably affordable and are considered of high quality in the state. For those sample PSUs for which a USPS list is unavailable or of insufficient quality, a listing of addresses can be obtained (if available) from property tax records. Alternatively, a listing of HUs can be made by the traditional listing method already described.

A sampling statistician should be consulted if more elaborate methods are required, such as geocoding addresses.

Secondary Sampling Unit Selection

When the average number of HUs per block is low (e.g., fewer than 20), it may not be necessary to choose a subsample of dwellings. It may be more practical to include all dwellings in the SSU sample. The cutoff for identifying sample blocks not requiring subsampling depends on the targeted average number of HUs per sample PSU. With an average Census 2000 household count of about 490 for Alaska, and with 99% of BGs with at least 65 households, HU subsampling will likely be required in most BGs sampled for the AN ATS. On the other hand, if the survey area is largely rural, the number of households in each BG may be low.

In those sample blocks where a subsample of dwellings must be chosen, without-replacement simple random sampling or systematic sampling may be applied to the BG-specific frames. The number of selected HUs in this stage of sampling must account for sample attrition due to ineligibility (e.g., vacant dwelling) and other reasons for nonresponse (e.g., refusal, not at home) to result in the required number of participating households within PSUs.

Missed Dwellings and Multiple Housing Units Located at Single Unit Address

It is not unusual for a small number of HUs to have been overlooked during counting and listing; therefore, missed-structure linkage procedures have been designed to address undercoverage in the sampling frame. When a missed-structure linkage procedure is used to address HUs missing from SSU frames, AN ATS screeners may have to check for missed HUs between a selected HU and the next one listed on the enumeration list. The resulting inclusion of discovered HUs should follow certain rules if such HUs number 5 or more (e.g., if 5 to 9 HUs are found at a sample address, then 1 is randomly selected for the study; if 10 to 19 HUs are found, then 2 are selected; and so forth).

Screeners will also have to determine whether multiple households live at each sample address. The type of HU data being gathered will determine whether one or all of the households at multihousehold addresses should be randomly chosen. For instance, if questions on exposure to secondhand smoke require information on all persons living on the premises, no subsampling of households should be done at multihousehold addresses. Otherwise, it may be best to randomly choose one of the households at the address.

If either of these two problems is encountered, it will add another stage to sampling and create the need to compute subsampling selection probabilities. If subselection is done by simple random sampling, the subsampling selection probability is simply the ratio of the number selected, divided by the number from which the subsample is selected.

4.2.4 Selection of Persons to Interview

Some special considerations apply to selecting and interviewing several eligible members from a single household. The benefits include an opportunity to reduce interviewer costs by requiring fewer household visits to reach the sample size targeted. Another advantage is that multiple selections from single households would provide for household-level estimates for tobacco use, which would in turn enable researchers to estimate the proportion of variance attributed to the variability in estimates at the HU level. The primary disadvantage, however, is that overall tobacco-use estimates for the state would be less precise because of cluster size increases. Consequently, recommended practice is that a single member be selected for participation from each eligible household.

It is helpful to consider households as clusters of individuals; that is, for this study, they are clusters of Alaska Native adults. One resident is randomly chosen for the survey interview in each household with at least one eligible Alaska Native resident. Although several alternative methods exist for randomly choosing the adult resident, the In-Person Screener for Selection of Eligible Household Respondent employs the "*n*th-oldest adult" approach. This approach is relatively easy to use and is generally noninvasive, especially as compared with the household roster approach, though it can somewhat skew the sample.[5]

In its simplest version, the *n*th-oldest adult approach begins by determining the number of eligible adults residing in the household and then chooses a random number between 1 and the number of reported residents. The selected resident is designated by age, relative to the oldest resident. For example, if there are three eligible adults and the number 2 is randomly chosen, then the second-oldest adult is selected for interview. To avoid selection bias, the interviewer is not allowed to substitute another eligible adult for the one that is randomly selected.

The problem with the *n*th-oldest, next/last-birthday, and other respondent-selection methods that choose a resident at random is that they often lead to a sex bias favoring females in the composition of the final respondent sample if the sex of the selected resident is not specified. For example, populations with 50:50 splits between males and females can lead to 40:60 or even 30:70 splits in the respondent sample. One reason for this sex imbalance is that, all else being constant, females are more likely than males to be available for and respond to interview surveys. Another explanation for this imbalance is the tendency for the household resident completing the In-Person Screener for Selection of Eligible Household Respondent (more likely female than male) to claim to be the selected respondent if the selection method does not explicitly indicate who is to be selected (Carr & Hertvik, 1993; Oldendick, Bishop, Sorenson, & Tuchfarber, 1988).

---

[5]Some surveys request specific, identifying information (e.g., the selected resident's first name or gender and age) to form a detailed household roster to use as the basis for resident selection. This method is preferred from a technical standpoint to reduce gender bias, but asking for more clearly identifying information on a household roster in this way increasingly has been seen by respondents as prying or intrusive and has led to higher refusal rates. The AN ATS Screener does not use this method.

Sex bias can be reduced by more explicitly specifying who is selected; therefore, the AN ATS member selection should specifically state the sex of the member to be surveyed. The In-Person Screener for Selection of Eligible Household Respondent asks for the number of adult Alaska Native males and adult Alaska Native females in the household. The interviewer can, for example, ask for the oldest female. With this approach, it is typical to require a separate random (i.e., Poisson) sampling decision for each household member, using selection probabilities that vary by subgroup characteristic (Lohr, 1999). Including sex as one of the control variables in the calibration (or poststratification) step for sample weights is another way to reduce the effect of sex bias.

The probability of inclusion for any sample member in multistage designs is the product of selection probabilities for sample outcomes in each stage that led to selecting that member; therefore, good records must be kept of the sampling process in each stage so that overall selection probabilities can be readily determined. When pencil-and-paper methods are used for in-person screening, the within-household sampling protocol must be followed carefully. The In-Person Screener for Selection of Eligible Household Respondent provides a clear, easy-to-follow protocol for deciding what n is when it asks for the nth-oldest adult, man or woman.

3   Weighting Methods

During analysis, formulas are applied to sample data to produce estimates of the population characteristics. Although the sample weight formulation for a community-list-based design differs from that of area sampling, the same sample weight adjustments apply to both designs. In addition, the statistical quality (or accuracy) of any survey estimate is measured by the size of its mean-squared error, which jointly depends on the precision (measured by variance or standard error of the estimate) and the bias of the estimate. Statistical inference based on probability samples offers an added advantage over inference using nonprobability samples: the analyst, using data from the sample selected, can directly obtain measures of the statistical precision of estimates, although, like the survey estimates, these measures of precision are also estimates. These precision measures are required in order to produce confidence intervals, tests of hypotheses, and other statistical products of analysis. To supplement efforts called for by the survey design, the bias of survey estimates must be measured when resources permit.

Appropriately estimating population characteristics and their precision requires that design features such as stratification, cluster sampling, and numerical measures of variable selection probabilities (i.e., leading to the computation of sample weights) be accommodated in analysis. Lohr (1999) offers a relatively recent review of the general design strategies and estimation issues related to sampling from finite populations. The representativeness of the selected sample may be altered by limitations in the selection and data-gathering processes, including frames that selectively cover the target population, and differential nonresponse by members of the selected sample and among data items sought from responding sample members (Lessler & Kalsbeek, 1992).

4.3.1 Sample Weights

To produce representative findings, the analyst should (1) compute sample weights to account for the process of sample selection and important composition-altering forces at work on the sample during the sampling and data collection processes, and (2) in analysis use statistical formulations that utilize these weights and appropriately account for stratification and cluster sampling in generating survey findings.

A sample weight is a number linked to a data record for any survey respondent. In general terms, it is computed as the inverse of the adjusted probability of obtaining the data for the respondent. An important component of this probability is the respondent's original selection probability based on the sample design. The inverse selection probability, or base weight, is often adjusted to account for unintended sample imbalance arising when the survey is conducted. More than one weight adjustment may be applied, and all are multiplicative.

Unless a weight is subsequently rescaled for analytic purposes (e.g., normalized to sum to the number of sample respondents), its value can be interpreted as an indication of the number of population members represented by the respondent. Separate sets of weights may be necessary when data are gathered for different types of data items associated with the respondent. For example, if data in a household survey are gathered for the selected households and for one resident chosen at random in each of those households, a separate set of weights is produced for the household data and the resident data.

If any of these sample weighting procedures requires clarification or elaboration, a sampling statistician should be consulted.

4.3.2 Weight Calculation

Some combination of the following steps is typically followed to produce a set of weights from a probability sample for the "*i*th" individual-respondent data record, with the final adjusted weight being the product of the value generated in each step. Assuming the availability of the needed information, the following weights and adjustments can be developed:

1. Base weight (determined by the probability of choosing the household and the method of respondent selection within the household).

2. Adjustment for nonresponse (to partially offset the biasing effects of differential response rates in the sample).

3. Adjustment for incomplete sample coverage (to partially correct for any bias due to differential coverage of the population by the list or lists from which the sample is chosen).

4. Adjustment to control variation among weights (to limit the loss in the precision of survey estimates due to widely variable sample weights).

5. Adjustment to calibrate the weights to the sampled population (to compensate for any sample imbalance not accommodated by the other adjustments).

Step 1 should always be completed in AN ATS samples. If all members on community lists or in the area surveyed are included in the survey, then the base weight is equaled to 1. If all members are not included with certainty, then the sample design must qualify as a probability sample design. Hence, steps followed in selecting the sample must be well documented so that exact selection probabilities can be determined for each survey respondent. Step 2 should be done if the sample has been divided into subgroups among which survey response rates differ. Step 3 is required when any evidence exists that the sampling frame did not cover the whole target population. Otherwise this adjustment is equaled to 1. Step 4 is particularly important in sites where the sample is significantly disproportionate (e.g., as a result of efforts to oversample Alaska Native households). This factor is equaled to 1 when weights are stable and truncation is not required. Step 5 adjusts the distribution of the sample based on the prior weighting steps to the distribution of the target population by demographic characteristics known to be correlated with tobacco use. This adjustment is 1 when no poststratification is done or when no reliable external data are available for calibration. The final statistical analysis weights are the product of all five weight components for the list sample or for the area sample.

4.3.3 Lack of Known Totals to Calibrate Weights

Step 5, sometimes referred to as "weighting up to known totals," or poststratification calibration is a final correction that helps make the weighted data more representative of the target population. Weights calibration, however, requires high-quality external data on the target population distribution by population characteristics highly correlated with adult tobacco use (e.g., sex, age, education). Large, national-level population surveys commonly rely on information obtained from the most recent decennial Census, the Current Population Survey, or the American Community Survey. Except for a statewide survey, finding a data source sufficiently current and of high quality to use in calibrating weights for a specific target population can be difficult. Although Census counts may not be current, data from the most recent decennial Census are usually the best available option.

4.4 Statistical Software for Complex Survey Designs

The sampling approaches for the AN ATS are complex in that they involve cluster selection, sampling stratification, and sample weights. Statistical software packages often used to select probability samples from list frames include Excel, SPSS and SAS (i.e., proc surveyselect). To prepare weights and weighted estimates from complex designs, one does best to use statistical software packages that rely on approximation or replication-based methods to estimate the variance of estimates (Wolter, 1985). A listing and several reviews of computer software that accommodates the sample design in this way are available online from the Survey Research Methods Section of the American Statistical Association (n.d.).

□.   □□□□□□□□ □□ □□□□□□□G

Interviewer training helps ensure that the data collected are accurate, complete, and consistent. The Alaska Native Adult Tobacco Survey (AN ATS) interviewer training program was developed to train interviewers specifically for the AN ATS. The full □a□□a □ative □dult □□□a□□□Survey □tervie□er □raining □anual is provided (Appendix I). The agenda and training manual can be adapted to specific circumstances, but no parts of the training program should be omitted.

□1   □he □la□□a □ati□e □□ult □□a□□□Sur□e□□nter□e□er □raining □anual

The Alaska Native Adult Tobacco Interviewer Training Manual comprises five sections:

- The Importance of Interviewers

- Ready Yourself for the Interview

- Know How to Conduct the Interview Successfully

- Practice Gaining Respondents' Cooperation

- Finally, Conduct the Interview

The manual focuses on administering the AN ATS, with emphasis on cultural sensitivity and refusal avoidance. The training program and manual should be supplemented with specific details about site-specific protocols that the interviewers should observe (i.e., maintaining and submitting timesheets, obtaining survey materials and supplies).

□.□   □reparati□n □□r □nter□e□er □raining

Thorough preparation is required to ensure that training sessions proceed as planned. The following hints will help avoid problems on the day of training and improve the effectiveness of the training:

- The training should be scheduled to occur shortly before the interviewing begins. Interviewers will forget much of what they learn if too much time elapses between the training and interviewing.

- The training should be scheduled to occur after all decisions have been made about the questionnaire and survey protocols. The training materials must reflect precisely how the interviewers are supposed to perform their work and how the materials will appear. It is confusing to tell interviewers that something will be different when they actually go to perform interviews.

- Sufficient time should be scheduled for the training. Most people are surprised at how long it takes to properly train interviewers and give them adequate practice with the survey protocols. There should be breaks every hour and a half to give interviewers time to stretch, use the facilities, get some water, and the like.

- Planning should ensure adequate space and facilities for the training. The facilities should accommodate all the interviewers comfortably, and interviewers should be able to see any presentation materials that are projected to the front of the room. The training rooms should be a comfortable temperature to help interviewers remain attentive.

- Arrangements should be made in advance for materials, parking, meals, and other logistics. For example, it is a good idea to plan on serving lunch at the training facility so that everyone is present when training classes begin. Adequate parking, likewise, helps ensure everyone is present and on time. There should be an adequate number of copies of handout materials for the interviewers and trainers.

- The trainers should be trained. Trainers must be thoroughly familiar with the training materials as well as the logistical plans for the training sessions. The trainers should not be responsible for logistics such as meals because such duties would take them away from their primary job of training the interviewers and being available to answer questions.

- Plans should be made for quizzing interviewers after training. All interviewers should be able to successfully complete a brief quiz after the training. Interviewers who cannot do so should be released from service or provided additional training.

5.3   Agenda for Training

Ideally, training should span 2 days so that every part of the training manual can be taught, with time allowed for practice and evaluation. A suggested agenda for the training follows.

5.1.1 Training Day 1

Introduction. Many experienced trainers find it valuable to have one of the principal researchers speak to interviewers at the opening of training. Interviewers who understand the purpose and importance of the research often do a better job of collecting quality data. At minimum, the instructor should begin by briefly explaining the purpose of the AN ATS for the particular community or village in which it will be conducted.

Questionnaire. The instructor reads the AN ATS, question by question, detailing how to record responses and reviewing the skip patterns attending particular clusters of questions.

Survey materials. The instructor reads and explains all the forms that will be used by interviewers. Forms include the Advance Letter, the Household Screener, the Informed Consent form, the "Sorry I Missed You" card, and the Receipt. The survey may have additional forms customized to this administration, and these should also be reviewed.

Objectivity and consistency. In the context of cultural sensitivity, the instructor explains the importance of the interviewer's objectivity and consistency. Objectivity in this context means that the interviewer maintains a neutral tone of voice and avoids words or actions that may imply approval or disapproval. *Consistency* is fundamental to data quality. Methods of survey administration must be consistent across all the work performed by a single interviewer, as well as across all interviewers. Interviewers are taught to avoid changing any words, to avoid providing ad hoc explanations of questions, and to observe similar safeguards.

Question-by-questions. The instructor reviews the question-by-questions, which guide interviewers in asking the interview questions, in probing for codable responses, and in answering any of the respondent's questions.

Frequently asked questions (FAQs). The survey sponsor may develop one or two pages listing answers to questions that respondents are likely to ask. The instructor reviews the answers so that all interviewers offer the same answers to the same questions. Interviewers are instructed not to provide ad hoc answers to questions. If a respondent asks a question that the interviewer is not trained to answer, the interviewer should refer the question to his or her supervisor. A sample set of FAQs has been attached to the *Interviewer Training Manual* (Attachment H-1). The answers in the sample must be modified to reflect circumstances surrounding the specific survey administration.

Confidentiality. The instructor discusses the importance of maintaining the confidentiality of all survey information, including not only the participant's interview responses, but also the participant's name, his or her address, and any personal information about the participant that the interviewer may learn or observe while in the participant's home.

Dress and demeanor. The instructor discusses the dress and demeanor appropriate for the community where the AN ATS is being conducted.

Time management. Issues of time management are addressed. In addition to teaching basic techniques for staying on schedule, the instructor imparts culturally appropriate methods for pacing the interview, for minimizing time spent socializing, and the like.

5.1.2 Training Day 2

Role-playing. Each interviewer administers the questionnaire to other interviewers. Partners are alternated so that interviewers are able to interview a wide variety of "respondents."

Observation. The instructor circulates during interviewing practice, providing each interviewer assistance, reinforcement, and constructive feedback.

Evaluation. Each trainee administers the questionnaire to the instructor (or other knowledgeable survey staff). In addition, the instructor asks the interviewer questions to determine whether the interviewer recalls the key parts of the training. Trainees who fail to show readiness to be interviewers after the 2 days of training should receive additional training or not serve in this role.

Paperwork. Interviewers selected to serve review the procedures for completing timesheets, accounting for incentive payments, retrieving materials, and returning completed questionnaires. This training module will be specific to the survey sponsor or survey organization.

6. ENHANCING RESPONSE RATES

Survey researchers are well aware of the importance of achieving the high response rates critical to establishing the reliability and accuracy of survey findings. Many well-known methods exist for doing so (American Association of Public Opinion Research, 2006–2007). Focus on the experience of researchers who have surveyed Alaska Native population distills lessons on improving response rates specifically for the Alaska Native Adult Tobacco Survey (AN ATS).

6.1 Benefitting From Experience

Survey response rates consistently have declined over the past 20 years across all segments of the population. Rigorous quantitative analysis to identify reasons for nonresponse, as well as what to do about it, is difficult because usually little is known about the nonrespondents. What is known about effective techniques is often based on qualitative review of call history records and interviewers' impressions of the relative success they have using different approaches. It is therefore recommended that any survey team include researchers and interviewers who have worked with the target population previously.

6.2 Using the Alaska Native Adult Tobacco Survey

Seasoned survey researchers generally affirm that using approaches sensitive to the specific cultural and social context of the target population will help achieve the highest rates possible. The foremost method for improving response rates among the Alaska Native population is, therefore, the use of the AN ATS itself. The survey design and the questionnaire were carefully developed to be sensitive to the specific cultural and social contexts of Alaska Native populations in the United States. The better the respondents can relate to the survey—the introduction, the questions, their communications with the interviewer—the more likely they are to cooperate and complete the interview.

6.3 Understanding the Survey Participants

Understanding one's survey participants is an important step in preparing a culturally sensitive survey program and protocol. Appended to this AN ATS Guidance Document is the AN ATS Cognitive Report Highlights (Appendix G). The highlights describe the characteristics of different subpopulations among Alaska Natives. For example, because literacy levels among Alaska Natives vary widely, understanding the literacy level of specific subpopulations of survey participants is fundamental to preparing comprehensible instructions. Moreover, familiarity with specific terms also varies among different subpopulations: Participants who have resided in rural areas for most of their lives may be unfamiliar with the term cessation class because such classes have never been taught in their community. In addition to possible language usability issues, cultural practices should be noted. For example, rural areas may observe seasonal events, events like those constituting the fishing season or the crop season. Such events may inform scheduling by revealing the most likely and least likely times to find participants at home.

□□ □uil□ing □app□rt t□ □mpr□□e □el□p□n□e □ate□

Experienced survey researchers understand the importance of creating rapport with respondents in order to gain and maintain their cooperation. Reviewed here are critical points in the interaction with potential respondents and suggestions for managing these moments.

6.4.1 Introduction of the Interviewer to the Household

Each interview will begin with a knock on the door. Interviewers must be able and ready confidently to introduce themselves and the survey in order to put the household respondent at ease and engage his or her interest in survey participation.

6.4.2 Hearing and Responding to Questions and Objections

The success of an interviewer often depends on his or her ability to quickly perceive and respond to potential respondents' concerns. Interviewers should expect household members to ask questions and have objections. The interviewer should be ready with accurate, specific information responsive to the household member's concerns. The □a□□a □ative □dult □□□a□□□Survey □ntervie□er □raining □anual includes a sample set of answers to frequently asked questions (FAQs). This set of answers will should be modified to reflect the particular survey's circumstances. Interviewers should be familiar with these answers and able to respond readily to the respondent's questions.

Interviewers often make the mistake of overanswering questions. It is important for the interviewer carefully to listen to the respondent, identify his or her core concern, and target any response to the core concern. More often than not, the respondent has a specific concern that can be addressed succinctly. When an interviewer elaborates unnecessarily, he or she can raise concerns that the respondent did not have until the interviewer introduced them.

If a respondent asks a question not covered by the FAQ, the interviewer should not invent an answer. Instead, the interviewer should acknowledge the question, make sure he or she understands it, and promise to recontact the respondent with an answer.

6.4.3 Selection of a Household Member to Be Interviewed

The process of selecting a respondent from among household members may feel invasive and make household members uncomfortable. Household members may try to substitute one member for another if the selected respondent is not comfortable completing the interview. Wives may try to substitute themselves for their husband, saying, "He won't do a survey." At such a point, the interviewer must be ready to convince the household members that (1) their information is totally confidential and (2) the selected respondent is the only one who may respond. As a first step, it is helpful for the interviewer to inform the respondent that his or her concerns are understandable. The second step is to assure the respondent that the survey procedures protect participants' rights.

6.4.4 Reading the Informed Consent

The interviewer must review the informed consent and obtain the respondent's agreement before beginning the interview. Even though it is written to be understandable, the consent can be intimidating. It is important to take whatever time is necessary to go through the consent and explain it to the respondent. The interviewer should reassure the respondent that the consent is designed to protect his or her rights as a survey participant.

6.4.5 Scheduling Return Visits

Sometimes when a respondent asks the interviewer to return at a later time, the request is really a "soft" refusal. The interviewer should impress on the respondent that he or she will be back at the designated date and time. If the respondent has trouble deciding a good time, it is often effective for the interviewer to propose two times—for example, "I can be here at 10:00 a.m. tomorrow or at 6:00 p.m., whichever is more convenient for you."

6.5 Appropriate Response to Concerns

It is worthwhile for researchers administering the AN ATS to invest in developing effective answers for expected questions and to invest in training interviewers to use these answers when they respond to respondents' concerns. Answers to FAQs for the AN ATS are provided in the *Alaska Native Adult Tobacco Survey Interviewer Training Manual* (see Attachment H-1). These FAQs can be customized to the specific circumstances of each survey.

Once the data are collected for the Alaska Native Adult Tobacco Survey, they must be transferred to a standardized, electronic format. With use of one of the many statistical software products specifically designed for survey research, the data can then be analyzed. Developing the questionnaire to be stored in an electronic format requires five steps: (1) developing a codebook, (2) reviewing hard-copy questionnaires, (3) adding administrative data to the questionnaires, (4) key-entering the data, and (5) checking the key-entry of data.

□1   □e□el□ping a C□□e□□□□

Although several methods could guide the preparation of a codebook, one of the simplest is to begin with a blank survey. Each question in the survey pertains to an issue called a *varia□le□*which may be defined as any data item that can vary. Each variable, or question, is given a short name that reflects the meaning of the question. For example, *B□ay* could mean *□rt□day□*

The following question asks respondents what type of smoker they are; the name of the variable may be □□PS□□ The person constructing the codebook prints the name of the variable next to the question in the codebook as illustrated below.

TYPSMK   Not including ceremonial or sacred smoking, do you now smoke cigarettes every day, some days, or not at all?

Every day	(1)
Some days	(2)
Not at all	(3)
Refused	(99)

Every possible response in the survey has a number next to it. Because statistical programs for computers read numbers for analysis, the data-input staff will input numbers rather than words. For example, using our variable □□PS□□□the numeric codes for answers would be as follows:

$$1 = \text{Every day}$$
$$2 = \text{Some days}$$
$$3 = \text{Not at all}$$
$$99 = \text{Refused to answer}$$

Once each question has been given a name and each answer has been assigned a number, the database can be prepared. The exact format for the database will be dictated by the statistical package used. If Excel is used, for example, a spreadsheet would be created with the variable names as column headings and the questionnaire identification numbers as the row headings. The respondent's numeric answers would then be entered in the appropriate cell (Table 7-1).

□a□□e □-1.   Sample □i□pla□□□□ata□a□e □□r □ue□ti□hnaire □e□p□n□e□

□ue□ti□hnaire □□n□	□ear	□□□S□□□	S□□	□G□	□□□C	□□C□□□□
101	2008	1	1	25	2	5
102	2008	3	2	45	3	99

The codes for variables other than TYPSMK are as follows:

SEX

> 1 = Male
> 2 = Female
> 9 = Refused to answer

AGE

> Actual age (e.g., □□year□□□d is coded as 19)

EDUC

> 1 = No formal schooling
> 2 = Some formal schooling but no diploma or GED
> 3 = Diploma or GED
> 4 = Some college but no degree
> 5 = College degree

INCOME

> 01 = $0 to $10,000
> 02 = $10,001 to $15,000
> 03 = $15,001 to $20,000
> 04 = $20,001 to $25,000
> 05 = $25,001 to $30,000
> 06 = $30,001 to $35,000
> 07 = $35,001 to $40,000
> 08 = $40,001 to $45,000
> 09 = Greater than $45,000
> 77 = Don't know / not sure
> 99 = Refused to answer

□□□ □e□ie□ing □ar□-C□p□□ue□ti□hnaire□

Questionnaires should be reviewed for problems such as missing data, more responses than a question asks for, illegible handwriting, and other clerical errors or problems that may call into question what the interviewer meant to enter. The resolution process may be started by asking the interviewer whether the interviewer recalls what he or she meant to enter or what the respondent said. If recall does not resolve the issue, the next step is to determine whether the dated may be imputed. For example, if birth date is provided but age is missing, age can be imputed from the birth date and the date of interview. If these steps fail to resolve the issue, a standard set of rules should be in place to resolve such matters. For example, a rule may state that the first response entered will be used if two answers are provided. If a problem cannot be resolved by any of these means, consider coding the answer as "missing." It would be as if the respondent had never answered the question.

For convenience during the key-entry step, the reviewer may write the number code that corresponds with each answer in the margin of the questionnaire. The reviewers must carefully proof their work to ensure that the correct codes are recorded in the database.

3   Adding Administrative Data to the Questionnaire

The first page of the questionnaire provides a space for coding items such as Year, Interview Supervisor, Interviewer, and Survey Number. The Membership List Version has space for entering the ID number of the sampled individual. Standardized lists of numerical codes have to be developed for these items (i.e., interviewers and interviewer supervisors should be assigned distinct codes). In addition (and if possible), including a printed, unique control number on each questionnaire before it is given to an interviewer can be a helpful tracking tool.

Key-Entering Data

Each respondent's interview responses must be key-entered into the data sheet or database. Errors are common at this stage, but measures can be taken to minimize them. Having a well-qualified staff perform the key-entry is one such measure: Experience entering large amounts of data with a low error rate is a necessary position requirement for key-entry personnel. If possible, data should be entered twice so that the two versions of the database can be compared. Any discrepancies can then be checked. Another method of checking data is to compare about 10% of the keyed data items with responses written on the survey. If more than a few errors are found, 100% of the data items should be checked against their source.

Conducting Checks on the Keyed Data

The data analyst or statistician should run an initial frequency on all variables. A frequency distribution will quickly reveal the existence of any invalid values. More complicated checks can test whether responses are consistent. For example, a smoker should have responses for all the questions asked of smokers. After checks on keyed data are performed and all inconsistencies and irregularities are resolved, the data are ready for analysis.

8. ANALYSIS AND REPORTING

Surveillance of tobacco use and related attitudes, knowledge, and beliefs is key to promoting reductions in tobacco use among Alaska Natives. Research has shown that well-conducted tobacco surveys produce reliable and accurate findings. Over the years, epidemiologists have developed effective questions, scales, and indices for measuring tobacco behaviors, attitudes, and beliefs. With good sample design, survey methodology, and survey execution, results from the Alaska Native Adult Tobacco Survey (AN ATS) can improve the ability to track tobacco-use knowledge, attitudes, and beliefs in a target population.

Five examples of analysis and reporting are provided in this chapter (Sections 8.1 through 8.5):

8.1   Basic Ways to Describe Data

8.2   Tobacco Use Among Young Adults

8.3   Exposure to Secondhand Smoke

8.4   Smoking Cessation

8.5   Analyses Using Additional Data Sets

These examples were chosen because they directly speak to the Centers for Disease Control and Prevention's (CDC's) and the Office on Smoking and Health's goals to (1) reduce initiation, (2) reduce exposure to secondhand smoke among nonsmokers, and (3) increase cessation. For each of these three major goals, one can track survey data over time to assess the population of interest. Such assessment may consist of comparing this population with other populations, identifying necessary intervention programs, developing health messages and other social marketing communications, and tracking the effectiveness of programs.

The first example, "basic ways to describe data," explains how to build a percentage frequency distribution (e.g., determine what percentages of the men in the survey area smoke). This example also answers "how many" questions (e.g., how many male smokers are there in the survey area?).

The next four sections (8.2 through 8.5) provide examples of types of analyses that can be performed on the AN ATS data collected. Each section begins by identifying the topic and the variables used to address that topic. Variables are divided between "outcome" measures (the behavior to be explained) and "domain" measures (the factors used to predict the behavior). The variables are identified by question number from the AN ATS. The example analyses presented in Sections 8.2 through 8.5 illustrate what can be learned from the AN

ATS data, but they are not intended to be an exhaustive treatment of analysis and reporting possibilities for the AN ATS.

Several software packages are designed specifically to analyze survey data. When selecting a statistical software package, the survey team should consider the type of analyses planned, the capacity and capabilities of the computer with which the analyses will be conducted, and the programs the analyst/programmer is familiar with or prefers.

8.1   Analyzing Categorical Data

8.1.1 Frequency Distributions and Point Estimates

A *frequency distribution* is simply the number of times respondents gave particular answers. If an interviewer asks respondents for their sex, the frequency distribution is the number of people who said "male" and the number who said "female." Researchers usually construct percentage frequency distributions. For example, if 200 people were interviewed, and 80 said "male" while 120 said "female," the percentage frequency distribution would be 40% "male" and 60% "female."

So long as proper sampling techniques have been used, these percentages can be ascribed to the whole population in the surveyed area. For example, if the survey respondents comprised 40% males and 60% females, one could safely say that 40% of all the Alaska Native residents in the surveyed area are male and 60% are female. Because only 200 residents were interviewed, the exact percentage of men and women in the surveyed area may be slightly higher or lower. The statistical analyst can provide the range within which the actual percentage will likely fall (e.g., 38% to 42% of all the Alaska Natives in the surveyed area are male).

Often the AN ATS is conducted to learn how many people in a community smoke. It is important to know that number if the survey organization is, for example, planning to provide smoking cessation classes. The percentage frequency distribution can be used to answer questions that ask "how many." For example, if a survey finds that 35% of the respondents smoke, then this finding means that about 35% of the Alaska Natives in the surveyed area smoke. If 1,000 Alaska Natives resided in the surveyed area, then one could estimate about 350 to be smokers (35% * 1,000). These numbers are called *point estimates.* As with a percentage, though, the exact number may be a little higher or lower. The survey's analyst can provide a range within which the point estimate will likely fall (e.g., 325 to 375 of all the Alaska Natives in the surveyed area are smokers).

8.1.2 Two-Way Classifications, or "Crosstabs"

Knowledge about smokers is important for determining how to target smoking intervention programs. Using the examples already given, if one wants to know whether men and women are equally likely to be smokers, or whether men and women show different patterns (i.e., men are more likely to smoke than women), a percentage frequency distribution of smokers as opposed to nonsmokers will be required, one including only the respondents who identified themselves as men. The same is done for women, and then the two are compared (Table 8-1).

Table 8-1. Sample Crosstab of Men's and Women's Smoking Status

Smoking Status	Men		Women		Total	
	n	%	*n*	%	*n*	%
Smoker	40	50	20	17	60	30
Nonsmoker	40	50	100	83	140	70
Total	80	100	120	100	200	100

In the example given in Table 8-1, it is easy to see that men are much more likely to be smokers than women (50%, compared with 17%). The point estimates are important, also. In this example, for the whole target population of 1,000 persons, 200 men are smokers (400 men * 50%) and about 100 women are smokers (600 women * 17%).

If a smoking intervention program is being planned, then knowing the ages of the smokers will probably be important. A table like Table 8-2 could be built to help make the intervention age appropriate.

Table 8-2 Sample Crosstab of Smokers' and Nonsmokers' Ages

Age	Smokers		Nonsmokers		Total	
	n	%	*n*	%	*n*	%
Younger than 12	2	3	10	7	12	6
12 to 14	3	5	10	7	13	7
15 to 17	10	16	30	43	40	20
18 to 25	15	25	40	29	55	28
26 to 54	25	42	45	32	70	35
55 or older	5	8	5	4	10	5
Total	60	100	140	100	200	100

8.1.3 Use of Table Formats

As discussed, data values in a databases are often in a coded form, so a table comparing sex and smoking status may look like Table 8-3.

□a□le □-3.   Sm□□ing Statu□□□□e□p□h□ent□□□□Se□□□ata □alue □ea□ing□□

□□□S□□	Se□ 1	□	99
1			
2			
99			

Analysts and other readers will find it more helpful if the numeric values are replaced with meaningful labels, as in Table 8-4.

□a□le □-□.   Sm□□ing Statu□□□□e□p□h□ent□□□□Se□□□e□□ripti□e □ea□ing□□

□□pe □□□m□□er	Se□ Female	□ale	□e□□e□t□re□p□h□
Smoker			
Nonsmoker			
Refused to respond			

This example includes both a row and a column for "refused to respond." The percentage frequency distributions must account for nonresponse either by including specific rows and columns or by subtracting them from the denominator before making the percentage frequency distributions. The survey analyst will be able to advise which handling is most appropriate in any specific analysis.

Table titles are an important way to help audiences understand analyses. As reflected in the examples given here, the table title should clearly identify the domain (who is included in the table); "outcomes," or dependent variables; and the precondition or independent variable.

□.□   □□□a□□□ □□e □m□□ng □□ung □□ult□

Tobacco use among young adults is a critical item of information for crafting tobacco cessation and tobacco-use avoidance programs. This section describes some analyses that may be conducted to learn about tobacco use among young adults in a particular surveyed area. It addresses topics such as the current smoking status of young adults in the community, the number of cigarettes smoked daily, the age at which smoking started, the portion of respondents who chew tobacco, and the age at which chewing tobacco started.

Table 8-5 summarizes the questionnaire items that are used in the analysis tables (Tables 8-6 through 8-11).

Table 8-5. Data Native Adult Tobacco Survey Questions Referenced in Tables 8-6 Through 8-11

Variable	Table 8-6	Table 8-7	Table 8-8	Table 8-9	Table 8-10	Table 8-11
Outcomes	Q2, Q4, Q6	Q53, Q54, Q58	Q7, Q8	Q4	Q2, Q3	Q55, Q56
Domains	Q129	Q129	Q129	Q129	Q140	Q140

8.2.1 Example 1: Current Smoking Levels

The cross-sectional percentage of young adults who are current smokers reflects both initiation of regular tobacco use and smoking cessation as illustrated in Table 8-6.

Table 8-6. "Current," "Former," and "Never" Cigarette Smokers Among Alaska Natives Aged 18 to 24 (Percent)

Age	Smoking Status		
	Current Smoker	Former Smoker	Never Smoker
18 years			
19 years			
20 years			
21 years			
22 years			
23 years			
24 years			

The age range 18 to 24 years was chosen for the tables in this section because for most people late adolescence and early adulthood are a period of transition. Initiation of regular smoking and development of nicotine addiction occur most often during this age, whereas older adults are less likely to initiate regular tobacco use. Many young adults start smoking as they transition into postsecondary education or full-time employment. Many smokers also quit during this period: National quit rates among smokers in this age group are higher than those among older smokers (Centers for Disease Control and Prevention, 1990).

Table 8-6 shows current smoking prevalence (smoke now, every day, or some days) for Alaska Natives, stratified by age. The "smoke now, every day, or some days" question was asked only of respondents who first had indicated that they had smoked at least 100 cigarettes in their lifetime. A *Current smoker* is defined, therefore, as a person who has smoked at least 100 cigarettes in his or her lifetime and was smoking every day or some days at the time of survey.

Differences in the initiation of smoking and early adulthood smoking have been shown to be related to numerous variables—sociodemographic, environmental, historical, behavioral, personal, and psychological (Centers for Disease Control and Prevention, 1998). If a survey has a sufficient sample size, additional analyses can be developed to explore associations between these variables and differences in smoking habits among the youth in the target population.

The AN ATS provides the data necessary to assess use of two tobacco products with growing popularity among youths—chewing tobacco and snuff. Table 8-7 illustrates a cross-sectional table displaying percentages of young adults who currently use chewing tobacco in order to reflect both initiation of regular use of chewing tobacco and cessation.

Table 8-7 "Current," "Former," and "Never" Chewing Tobacco Users Among Alaska Natives, Ages 18 to 24 (Percent)

	Chewing tobacco status		
Age	**Current user**	**Former user**	**Never user**
18 years			
19 years			
20 years			
21 years			
22 years			
23 years			
24 years			

As with cigarette smoking, the age range 18 to 24 is a period of transition. Knowledge about initiation is important in designing effective intervention programs.

The extent of the adverse health effects of smoking is influenced by the intensity of the smoking. Table 8-8 provides one way to assess the potential adverse health effects among youths.

Table 8-8. **Number of Cigarettes Smoked Daily by "Every Day" and "Some Days" Smokers Among Alaska Natives Aged 18 to 24 (Percent)**

Age	Number of Cigarettes Smoked Daily			
	Less than 1	1–10	11–20	More than 20
18 years				
19 years				
20 years				
21 years				
22 years				
23 years				
24 years				

8.2.2 Example 2: Age at Initiation of Smoking

Progression to established smoking depends in part on the age at which people start experimenting with smoking. One good measure of progression to established smoking during adolescence is the cross-sectional prevalence of persons who by early adulthood had smoked at least 100 cigarettes, as illustrated in Table 8-9.

Table 8-9. **Earliest Age at Which Alaska Natives Aged 18 to 24 Smoked 100 Cigarettes (Percent)**

Age	Smoked 100 Cigarettes in lifetime	
	Yes	No
Younger than 12 years		
12 to 14 years		

The AN ATS is designed for administration to adults aged 18 or older. Therefore, this table is based on recall of those aged 18 to 24. The table could include older persons, but their recall may not be as good as that of younger persons. In addition, experiences of those 18 to 24 may reflect more current patterns in the progression to establish smoking.

By "progression to established smoking," we mean that people have advanced through the smoking uptake stages to the point that they are no longer "experimenters" (Mowery, Farrelly, Haviland, Gable, & Wells, 2004).

The AN ATS asks respondents to report the age at which they first tried a cigarette. Table 8-10 shows the age at which the respondent first tried a cigarette, by level of education completed, among those who were aged 30 years or older at survey.

△a△e △-1△. △ge at △hi△h △a△a △ati△e△△ge△3△ △r △l△er Fir△t Sm△△e△a Cigarette△△△△△u△ati△n △△er△ent△

△ighe△t e△u△ati△n le△el △△mplete△	Age △ir△t △m△△e△igarette					
	1△ △r △△unger	11–1△	1△–1△	1△–1△	19–△△	△1 △r △l△er
Less than high school						
High school graduate						
Some college						
College graduate						

As in Table 8-9, a problem with this measure is recall bias because older respondents, especially, may not accurately remember the age at which they first tried a cigarette. Nevertheless, the age of first experimentation with smoking remains an important indicator—one that helps focus interventions on the most appropriate age groups. An important tobacco control strategy has been to try to delay experimentation and regular smoking until late adolescence and early adulthood, a time when most people presumably have better skills and knowledge for rejecting tobacco use as an unhealthy practice. Level of education is appropriate for this table because most people have completed their formal education by age 30.

A similar analysis could be conducted to assess use of chewing tobacco and snuff, as illustrated in Table 8-11.

△a△e △-11. △ge at △hi△h △a△a △ati△e △ge△3△ △r △l△er Fir△t △egularl△△△e△ Che△ing △△△a△△△△△△u△ati△n △△er△ent△

△ighe△t e△u△ati△n le△el △△mplete△	△ge △ir△t regularl△△u△e△ △he△ing t△△a△△△					
	1△ △r △△unger	11–1△	1△–1△	1△–1△	19–△△	△1 △r △l△er
Less than high school						
High school graduate						
Some college						
College graduate						

The AN ATS does not ask about the age at which the respondent first used chewing tobacco; therefore, Table 8-11 uses age at first regular use as a proxy measure.

△3 △△p△△ure t△ Se△△n△han△ Sm△△e

Exposure to secondhand tobacco smoke causes lung cancer, other respiratory diseases, and coronary heart disease in adults; inhalation of tobacco smoke also causes symptoms such as runny nose and throat irritation (Centers for Disease Control and Prevention, 2006). Section 8.3 offers some variables for analysis of AN ATS data on exposure to secondhand smoke. These variables address topics such as exposure to secondhand smoke in the home, rules governing smoking in the home, the frequency with which people smoke in the home, the number of smokers in the home, workplace exposure, and attitudes toward prohibition of smoking.

Table 8-12 summarizes the variables used in the tables developed to study these topics (Tables 8-13 through 8-17).

Table 8-12. Data Native Adult Tobacco Survey Questions Referenced in Tables 8-13 through 8-17

Variable	Table 8-13	Table 8-14	Table 8-15	Table 8-16	Table 8-17
Outcomes	Q110	Q109	Q6, Q108	Q113	Q147, Q148
Domains	Q141	Q141	Q132	Q141	Q2, Q4, Q6

8.3.1 Example 1: Exposure to Secondhand Smoke at Home

Young children are particularly vulnerable to secondhand smoke in the home because they spend so much time there. Measurement of home exposure to secondhand smoke is accomplished by three means: ambient air monitoring, biological markers of exposure among people who live in the home, and self-reports of exposure. The AN ATS uses self-report, for which there are two questions: a question about home rules (Q110) and a question about recall of smoking in the home (Q109).

The percentage distribution of restrictions on family members' and guests' smoking in the home is shown in Table 8-13. These home rules are stratified by income level. The income-level groups can be adjusted to distribute the target population more evenly and meaningfully across the groups.

Table 8-13. Home Smoking Rules among Data Native Adults, Home (Percent)

Annual household income ($)	Smoking permitted inside the home			
	Not anywhere or at any time	Allowed some places or time	Allowed anywhere and at any time	Don't know
Less than 25K				
25K to less than 50K				
50K to less than 75K				
75K or more				

Although home rules can indicate exposure, they do not necessarily measure all secondhand smoke exposure at home, because smoking bans may be ignored. An alternative measure of home exposure among nonsmokers is possible with the AN ATS: Q109 asks for the number of days that someone, excluding the respondent, smoked in the home during the 7 days preceding the interview. Table 8-14 shows the percentage of persons who reported that someone other than the respondent smoked in the home during the 7 days preceding the interview, by income level.

Table 8-14. Number of Days in Past Week That Someone Smoked Inside Home, by Income (Percent)

Annual household income ($)	Number of days smoking occurred in home during past week			
	None	1–2	3–6	7
Less than 25K				
25K to less than 50K				
50K to less than 75K				
75K or more				

Table 8-14 illustrates one approach to estimating the number of nonsmokers in the survey area who are exposed to secondhand smoke in their homes. Some programming is required to create the table categories. First, one must subset those respondents who are nonsmokers. This subset is the denominator. Next, one must recode into appropriate groups the number of days that smoking occurred inside the home. Notably, Table 8-14 does not measure the prevalence of households in which people are exposed to secondhand smoke, because the AN ATS is generally weighted to the population of people, not households. Moreover, Table 8-14 does not include home exposure as identified by smoker respondents to the survey.

Research has shown that total number of smokers in a household has a stronger relationship with increased serum cotinine levels in children than the number of days someone smoked in the home does (Pirkle et al., 1996). A measure of children's potential exposure to secondhand smoke, based on the number of smokers in the home, is possible with the AN ATS. Information on whether the respondent is a smoker, combined with the smoking status of all other adults in the home, yields the number of smokers in the household. Table 8-15 shows the percentage of respondents who live in homes with one or more smokers, by the age of children in the home.

Table 8-15. Number of Adult Smokers in Home by Age of Children in Home (Percent)

Age of Children in home	Number of Smokers in home			
	None	1	2	More than 2
Newborn to 11 months old				
1–4 years old				
5–11 years old				
12–17 years old				

Notably, the outcome for Table 8-15 (number of adult smokers in the home) does not include adolescent smokers. In addition, the domain levels in Table 8-15 are not mutually exclusive. For example, a respondent who lives in a home with a newborn and a 5-year-old child will be counted in two rows of the table.

Even with these indicators, it is difficult to produce exact measures of exposure. Potential exposure as measured by the numbers of smokers in the home may not reflect actual exposure, because parents may choose not to smoke at home when their children are present. On the other hand, smoking at any time in the home may expose children after the fact because secondhand smoke tar is deposited on surfaces and evaporates as fine particles (Nazaroff & Singer, 2004). The levels of delayed exposure and risk from this exposure are as yet unknown.

8.3.2 Example 2: Exposure of Nonsmokers to Workplace Secondhand Smoke

The AN ATS asks respondents whether they recall anyone's smoking inside the building where they worked in the week preceding the survey (Q113). This question is asked only of respondents who are employed for wages or who are self-employed and work outside the home. Table 8-16 shows the incidence of workplace smoking by income level.

Table 8-16. Who's Workplace Exposure in the Past 7 Days or Past 4 Weeks Whether Smoking Is Permitted in Home (Percent)

Annual household income ($)	Workplace exposure in past 7 days (nonsmoker)	
	Yes	No
Less than 25K		
25K to less than 50K		
50K to less than 75K		
75K or more		

Occupational exposure to smoke poses a significant risk to nonsmokers. Waiters and waitresses, for example, may be continually exposed to smoke during their shifts.

Construction workers who share transportation to and from worksites in truck cabs have briefer but more concentrated exposure. The burden of exposure may fall more heavily on lower-income persons.

8.3.3 Example 3: Attitudes Toward Laws on Clean Indoor Air

Through ordinances and regulations, state and local governments may mandate that nonsmokers be protected from secondhand smoke. Public support for banning smoking in public places increased dramatically during the past 30 years.

The AN ATS contains a set of questions that measure respondents' support for smoking bans in indoor places. Two questions ask about attitudes toward smoking inside tribal or corporation buildings (Q147) and community centers (Q148). Table 8-17 can be used to assess support for smoking bans in these locations.

Table 8-17. Whether Native Adult Thinks Smoking Should Be Prohibited in Tribal or Corporation Buildings or Community Center, by Smoking Status (Percent)

	Thinks smoking should be prohibited in			
Smoking Status	All area of tribal corporation building	Some area of tribal corporation building	All area of community center	Some area of tribal corporation building
Current smoker				
Former smoker				
Never smoker				

Table 8-17 was constructed by appending two separate cross-tabulations, one for each question. Standard statistical analyses like chi-square tests cannot be performed with this data structure, which allows each respondent to be represented multiple times. It is possible to test for a difference in attitudes between one status and all others. For statistical methods for comparing two binomial proportions, see Fleiss, Levin, and Paik (2003).

8.4 Smoking Cessation

Information about smoking cessation is important to the crafting of intervention programs. Section 8.4 describes some analyses that may be conducted to learn how best to target smoking cessation efforts. This section addresses topics such as the readiness of smokers to quit, the methods smokers have already used to try to quit, and how successful smokers have been in quitting. Table 8-18 summarizes the variables used to conduct these analyses (Tables 8-19, 8-20, and 8-21).

Table 8-18. Data Tables Built from Survey Questions Presented in Tables 8-19 Through 8-21

Variable	Table 8-19	Table 8-20	Table 8-21
Outcomes	Q14, Q22, Q23	Q15, Q16, Q17, Q18, Q19, Q20	Q13
Domains	Q140 Q137[a]	Q130	Q129

[a] This question appears in the Member List Version of the questionnaire.

8.4.1 Example 1: Stages of Change

The AN ATS can be used to develop a stage-of-change index as illustrated in Table 8-19. The measure is based on a series of questions, including whether the respondent had made a quit attempt during the 12 months preceding the survey, readiness to quit in the next 6 months, and readiness to quit in the next 30 days.

Table 8-19. Alaska Native Current Smokers' Stage of Change Toward Smoking Cessation by Population Level (Percent)

Highest education level completed	Stage of Change toward Smoking Cessation			
	Precontemplation	Contemplation	Preparation	Action
Less than high school				
High school graduate				
Some college				
College graduate				

Respondents who at the time of interview were not seriously considering quitting in the next 6 months are "precontemplators" (Q22 = 2). Those who were seriously considering quitting in the next 6 months but not in the next 30 days are "contemplators" (Q22 = 1 and Q23 = 2 or 3). Those who were planning to quit in the next 30 days but who had not made a serious quit attempt in the past year are in the "preparation" stage (Q22 = 1, Q23 = 1, and Q14 = 2). Those smokers who were planning to quit in the next 30 days and who had made a quit attempt in the past year are in the "action" stage (Q22 = 1, Q23 = 1, and Q14 = 1). The stage-of-change index is constructed only for current smokers.

The delineation of stages of change as shown in Table 8-19 can be helpful in determining the best approach to take in smoking cessation programs. The stage of change is limited, though, in that it can measure only readiness to quit and cannot be used to infer actual quit attempts or success in quitting. Success in quitting depends on a host of other factors, including degree of addiction, level of self-efficacy for quitting, and level of self-confidence for quitting, as well as other environmental influences on individuals' smoking behaviors.

8.4.2 Example 2: Methods Used to Quit at Last Quit Attempt

Many therapies, self-help materials, and programs have been developed to assist individuals in quitting smoking. Table 8-20 shows the prevalence of use of the six quitting methods.

Table 8-20. Methods Used to Quit Smoking among Alaska Native Current and Former Smokers, by Sex (Percent)

Sex	Nicotine gum	Nicotine patch	Medication like Chantix	Cold turkey	Pledge	Stop Smoking Classes, call Quit line, or Counseling
Male						
Female						

On the AN ATS, the methods were asked about independently; respondents could choose more than one method. Use of medications, including nicotine replacement therapy, is asked about in Q15 and Q16. Q17 asks about using a medication like Zyban, Chantix, or nicotine lozenges. Q18 asks if the respondent went "cold turkey" (on his or her own). Q19 asks if the respondent used a prayer or took a pledge. Q20 asks if the respondent used any other type of help, such as stop-smoking classes, a telephone quit line, or counseling. These questions are asked of both current and former smokers. It is possible to test for a difference in prevalence of use between males and females. For statistical methods for comparing two binomial proportions, see Fleiss, Levin, and Paik (2003).

8.4.3 Example 3: Length of Abstinence Among Former Smokers

Smokers and ex-smokers typically report making multiple attempts to quit (Centers for Disease Control and Prevention, 1990). Among those who have quit for a single day, the failure rate is very high. The longer the quit attempt lasts, the more likely it is that the individual will successfully avoid relapsing. The length of abstinence is used as an indicator of smokers' overall success in quitting and an indirect measure of smokers' knowledge of resources to help them quit. Table 8-21 shows the length of abstinence for current and former smokers.

Table 8-21. Length of Abstinence Among Alaska Native Current and Former Smokers (Age Percent)

Age		Length of Abstinence		
	Up to 1 month	1–3 months	3 months to 1 year	Longer than 1 year
18–24 years				
25–44 years				
45–64 years				
65 years or older				

The outcome variable for Table 8-21 is a recode of Q13. The denominator for this table is persons who had smoked at least 100 cigarettes in their lifetime but were not smoking at time of interview (ascertained from Q2, Q4, and Q6). Respondents who reported in Q13 that they never smoked regularly are excluded from the denominator.

8.5 Use Additional Data Sets

Reviewing findings from other reputable tobacco-related studies and relating that information to the surveyed area can help inform the smoking reduction strategies to implement for that area. Section 8.5 presents two such analyses. The first looks at data for Alaska from the Tobacco Use Supplement (TUS) to the Current Population Survey (CPS; National Cancer Institute, 2010) to learn about occupational differences in Alaska's workplace smoking policies. The second compares AN ATS findings about people's beliefs in the harmfulness of secondhand smoke with the strength of local laws to ban indoor smoking in worksites and public places such as restaurants.

Table 8-22 summarizes the AN ATS variables used in the comparison presented in Table 8-24 (no AN ATS findings are presented in Table 8-23).

Table 8-22. Alaska Native Adult Tobacco Survey Questions Referenced in Tables 8-23 and 8-24

Variable	Table 8-23	Table 8-24
Outcomes	TUS-CPS	Q115
Domains	TUS-CPS	ANRF

Notes: TUS = Tobacco Use Supplement; CPS = Current Population Survey; ANRF = Americans for Nonsmokers' Rights Foundation.

8.5.1 Example 1: Occupational Differences in Workplace Smoking Policies

Differences in workplace policies among different groups can be explored by using the TUS-CPS. The TUS-CPS is a national survey that is prestratified by state (i.e., the sample is drawn independently within each state). Since the same respondents are asked both the

CPS and TUS questions, respondent and household occupational information (CPS) can be compared to tobacco-use data (TUS). There are enough completed interviews at the state level to make reliable individual state estimates for many domains. Although the surveyed area may cover only a part of Alaska, state-level data can provide useful information on cultural and environmental factors affecting smoking in the area.

Table 8-23 shows workplace smoking policies in Alaska by three broad occupational categories: white collar, blue collar, and food service.

☐a☐e ☐-☐3. ☐mpl☐☐e☐Sm☐☐er☐in ☐a☐☐a ☐h☐☐☐☐r☐in Sm☐☐e-Free☐Sm☐☐ng-☐l☐☐e☐☐an☐☐☐-☐☐i☐☐☐r☐pla☐e☐☐☐☐☐☐☐upati☐h ☐☐er☐ent☐

	☐☐r☐pla☐e ☐m☐☐ng p☐li☐☐		
☐☐☐upati☐nal ☐a☐☐	☐☐p☐li☐☐	Sm☐☐ng all☐☐e☐	Sm☐☐e-☐ree
White collar			
Blue collar			
Food service			

Notes: These respondents reported smoking every day during the year preceding the survey. The table excludes self-employed persons and persons who work outdoors.

Source: U.S. Census Bureau (2001–2007). Tobacco Use Supplement, Current Population Survey [Data files]. ☐ati☐nal ☐an☐er ☐☐☐titute ri☐☐☐a☐☐☐r ☐☐nit☐ring and ☐et☐☐d☐☐☐e☐☐te☐Retrieved February 24, 2009, from http://riskfactor.cancer.gov/studies/tus-cps/info.html.

Although many business organizations have adopted smoke-free worksite policies, certain industries lag behind, particularly food service establishments and bars that serve the public (Shopland, Anderson, Burns, & Gerlach, 2004). Servers and other food service workers are often exposed to secondhand tobacco smoke while working. The occupational categories shown in Table 8-23 are a recode based on the detailed occupational codes used by the CPS (U.S. Census Bureau, 2008). The TUS-CPS is sponsored by the National Cancer Institute and is fielded every 3 years.

8.5.2 Example 2: Merging Alaska Native Adult Tobacco Survey Data with Environmental Data

The AN ATS can be used to assess differences in attitudes and beliefs about exposure to secondhand smoke and to determine whether the respondent lives in a locality with a law on clean indoor air. Information on the strength of local laws mandating clean indoor air is available from the Americans for Nonsmokers' Rights Foundation (ANRF; American Nonsmokers' Rights Foundation, 2010b). Since 1985 ANRF has tracked, collected, and analyzed local tobacco control ordinances, bylaws, and Board of Health regulations (American Nonsmokers' Rights Foundation, 2010a). Each ordinance database record has more than 200 fields detailing characteristics of the law or regulation for each municipality.

Table 8-24 uses one of the primary fields in the ANRF database: whether the local ordinance completely bans smoking in public indoor places, whether the local ordinance is qualified (meaning that the ordinance exempts certain indoor places), or whether the local ordinance is weak or nonexistent. Information on the strength of local laws can be merged into the AN ATS by zip code of the targeted population. Information on local ordinances for a specific state can be obtained by contractual agreement with ANRF.

Q115 asks respondents whether they think that breathing secondhand smoke is harmful to one's health. This question is the outcome for Table 8-24.

Table 8-24. Belief about the Harmful Effect of Breathing Secondhand Smoke by Strength of Local Clean Indoor Air Law (Percent)

Strength of local law on clean indoor air	Belief about breathing secondhand smoke		
	Harmful to one's health	Not harmful at all to one's health	Don't know
100% ban[a]			
Qualified[b]			
Weak or no law			

[a] Law prohibits smoking in all worksites and all public indoor places, including restaurants and freestanding bars.
[b] Law allows exemptions for some indoor places.

As of October 2009, 71% of the U.S. population lived in areas that ban smoking in workplaces, restaurants, or bars. A total of 3,117 municipalities in the United States have local laws in effect that restrict where smoking is allowed. Thirty-eight states and the District of Columbia have local laws in effect that require 100% smoke-free workplaces, restaurants, or bars (American Nonsmokers' Rights Foundation, 2010c).

Alaska statewide smoking law generally requires the designation of smoking and nonsmoking areas and warning signage in most enclosed workplaces and public places. Smoking is specifically prohibited in (1) schools, (2) meetings of state or local government public bodies, (3) health care facilities, and (4) elevators (Alaska Stat. §§ 18.35.300–18.35.330). Warning signage must be posted in a number of other locations, such as workplaces, government offices, universities, adult daycare facilities, courtrooms, restaurants that seat more than 50 people, and correctional facilities.

Localities in Alaska with smoking bans that include all bars and restaurants are as follows:

- Anchorage banned smoking in all enclosed workplaces, including bars, restaurants, and private clubs ("Anchorage voters embrace smoking ban," 2007, April 7).

- Juneau banned smoking in all bars, restaurants, and private clubs (American Nonsmokers' Rights Foundation, 2010c).

- Klawock banned smoking in all enclosed workplaces, including bars and restaurants (American Nonsmokers' Rights Foundation, 2010c).

Localities in Alaska with smoking bans that do not include all bars and restaurants are as follows (American Nonsmokers' Rights Foundation, 2010c):

- Barrow banned smoking in all restaurants, but not bars or all other workplaces.

- Dillingham banned smoking in all restaurants, but not bars or all other workplaces.

- Fairbanks banned smoking in all workplaces, excluding bars and restaurants.

- Sitka banned smoking in all enclosed workplaces, including restaurants but exempting bars.

Use of other findings may extend beyond the findings of the TUS-CPS or the ANRF. For example, CDC's *Tobacco Control State Highlights* for Alaska (Centers for Disease Control and Prevention, 2010) provides information on a broad range of comparative and contextual topics, such as the following:

- Average Annual Smoking-Attributable Mortality, 1997–2001
  - Average Annual Smoking-Attributable Productivity Losses, 1997–2001
  - Smoking-Attributable Expenditures, 1998
  - Adult Cigarette Use, 2006
  - Adult Attempts to Quit Smoking, 2006
- Tobacco-Related Disparities in Cigarette Use Among Adult Population Groups, 2006
- Youth Cigarette Use
  - Youth Attempts to Quit Smoking
  - Smoke-Free Home Rules, 2003
  - Smoke-Free Worksite Rules, 2003
  - Smoke-Free Indoor Air Legislation, 2007
  - Excise Tax Legislation, 2007
  - Licensure Legislation, 2007
  - Advertising Legislation, 2007
  - Youth Access Legislation, 2007
  - Preemption Legislation, 2007
  - State Revenue From Tobacco Sales and Settlement
  - Federal and National Investment in Tobacco Control, 2006

Other informational sources include surveys mentioned earlier in the context of questionnaire design: the Behavioral Risk Factor Surveillance System, the National Health and Nutrition Examination Survey, and the National Health Interview Survey.

9.   REFERENCES AND RESOURCES

9.1   Introduction

American Nonsmokers' Rights Foundation (2010b). *American nonsmokers' rights.* Retrieved June 8, 2010, from http://no-smoke.org/index.php

Centers for Disease Control and Prevention (2004). *The health consequences of smoking: A report of the Surgeon General.* Atlanta, GA: Author.

Kaufert, J. M., O'Neil, J. D., & Koolage, W. W. (1991). The cultural and political context of informed consent for Native Canadians. *Arctic Medical Research Suppl,* 181–184.

This article presents a case study.

Kincaid, J. P., Fishburne, R. P., Rogers, R. L., & Chissom, B. S. (1975). *Derivation of new readability formulas (automated readability index, fog count and flesch reading ease formula) for Navy enlisted personnel*: Naval Air Station, Memphis, TN.

Norton, I. M., & Manson, S. M. (1996). Research in American Indian and Alaska Native communities: Navigating the cultural universe of values and process. *Journal of Consulting and Clinical Psychology, (5),* 856–860.

This article offers guidance on defining the population of American Indians and Alaska Natives for inclusion in a survey, enhancing participation of the tribes, and obtaining approval from the institutional review board; in addition, it discusses issues of confidentiality and anonymity of individuals and tribes.

Piquemal, N. (2001). Free and informed consent in research involving Native American communities. *American Indian Culture and Research Journal, (1),* 65–79.

This article offers recommendations for negotiating responsibilities before seeking consent, obtaining consent from relevant authorities, reconfirming consent as work proceeds, and providing the community with data.

9.2   Survey Instruments and Supporting Materials

Centers for Disease Control and Prevention, National Center for Health Statistics. (2008). *National Health and Nutrition Examination Survey.* Retrieved February 14, 2009, from http://www.cdc.gov/nchs/about/major/nhanes/intro_mec.htm

Centers for Disease Control and Prevention, National Centers for Health Statistics. (2008). National Health Interview Survey tobacco information Web site. Retrieved February 14, 2009, from http://www.cdc.gov/nchs/about/major/nhis/tobacco/nhis_tobhoma.htm

Centers for Disease Control and Prevention. (2009). The Behavioral Risk Factor Surveillance System. Retrieved February 14, 2009, from http://www.cdc.gov/brfss/

Dillman, D. A. (2000). *Mail and internet surveys: The tailored design method.* New York: Wiley.

9.3   Sampling and Weighting

American Statistical Association, Survey Research Methods Section. (n.d.). Summary of Survey Analysis Software. Retrieved July 6, 2010, from http://www.hcp.med.harvard.edu/statistics/survey-soft/.

Carr, K., & Hertvik, J. (1993). □it□n□□□u□e□□□d □ele□ti□n□□□any□□dy li□tening□Paper presented at the Proceedings of the Section on Survey Research Methods, American Statistical Association.

This conference paper covers techniques for survey sampling.

Cochran, W. G. (1977). *Sa□□ing te□□hi□ue□*(3rd ed.). New York: Wiley.

This book offers a general review of sampling techniques and includes general techniques for survey sampling.

Kalsbeek, W. D. (2003). Sampling minority groups in health surveys. *Stati□ti□□in □edi□ne□* □□, 1527–1549.

This article offers a general review of survey sampling techniques.

Kalton, G., & Maligalig, D. S. (1991). A comparison of methods of weighting adjustment for nonresponse. In *Pr□□eeding□□□t□e □□□□□hnual □e□ear□□□□h□ren□e*. Washington, DC: U.S. Bureau of the Census.

This conference paper reviews some common nonresponse models and weighting adjustment procedures.

Kish, L. (1965). *Survey □a□□□ing*. New York: Wiley.

This book offers general techniques for survey sampling.

Kish, L. (1995). *Survey □a□□□ing*. New York: Wiley-Interscience.

This classic, accessible book offers techniques for survey sampling.

Lessler, J. T., & Kalsbeek, W. D. (1992). □□n□a□□□ing err□r in □urvey□ New York: Wiley.

This book offers techniques for measuring nonsampling error.

Oldendick, R. W., Bishop, G. F., Sorenson, S. B., & Tuchfarber, A. J. (1988). A comparison of the Kish and last birthday methods of respondent selection in telephone surveys. *□□□rnal □□□□□□□al Stati□ti□□□□*(4), 307–318.

This article offers techniques for survey sampling.

SAS Institute. (2007). *S□S□S□□□□□□u□er□guide*. Cary, NC: Author.

This manual offers guidance to the computer application for statistical processing.

Srinath, K. P. (1996). *Sa□□e all□□ati□n and □ele□ti□n □et□□d□□□r □ver□a□□ing □□□□□□□u□lati□n□* Salt Lake City, UT: American Association for Public Opinion Research.

This paper presents techniques for improving subpopulation estimates by keeping the strata sample sizes close to the sample sizes considered optimum from the viewpoint of efficiency of the overall estimates.

U.S. Census Bureau. (n.d.). Census 2000 geographic terms and concepts. Retrieved July 6, 2010, from http://www.census.gov/geo/www/tiger/glossry2.pdf.

Wolter, K. M. (1985). *□ntr□du□ti□n t□varian□e e□ti□ati□n*. New York: Springer-Verlag.

This book offers techniques for estimating variance.

9.☐ Enhancing Response Rates

American Association of Public Opinion Research. (2006–2007). Resources for researchers. Retrieved February 14, 2009, from http://www.aapor.org/resources

> This Web page offers general techniques for enhancing response rates.

Delener, N. (1995). An integrative review of nonresponse errors in survey research. Research in Marketing, 49–80.

> This article identifies major sources of nonresponse error and strategies for nonresponse error reduction.

Edwards, S., Slattery, M. L., Mori, M., Berry, T. D., Caan, B. J., Palmer, P., et al. (1994). Objective system for interviewer performance evaluation for use in epidemiologic studies. American Journal of Epidemiology(11), 1020–1028.

> This article presents a system for evaluating interviewer performance in epidemiologic studies.

Groves, R. (2002). Survey nonresponse. New York: Wiley.

> This book reviews the current state of research and practice for survey nonresponse.

Macedo, J., Reano, L., Weber, J., & Easton, A. (2004). Strategies for surveying American Indian and Alaska Native communities. In Proceedings Statistics Canada International Symposium. Ottawa, Ontario: Statistics Canada.

> This paper from the Symposium 2004: Innovative Methods for Surveying Difficult-to-reach Populations offers findings of a Centers for Disease Control and Prevention panel with survey experts and tribal representatives; it concerns surveys conducted involving American Indian and Alaska Native adult tobacco questionnaires.

Yu, J., & Cooper, H. (1983). A quantitative review of research design effects on response rates to questionnaires. Journal of Marketing Research, 36–44.

> This article reviews techniques used to increase response rates.

9.☐ Informed Consent

Kaufert, J. M., O'Neil, J. D., & Koolage, W. W. (1991). The cultural and political context of informed consent for Native Canadians. Arctic Medical Research Suppl, 181–184.

> This article presents a case study.

Kincaid, J. P., Fishburne, R. P., Rogers, R. L., & Chissom, B. S. (1975). Derivation the readability formula automated readability index fog count and flesch reading ease formula for navy enlisted personnel. Memphis, TN: Naval Air Station.

Norton, I. M., & Manson, S. M. (1996). Research in American Indian and Alaska Native communities: Navigating the cultural universe of values and process. Journal of Consulting and Clinical Psychology(5), 856–860.

> This article offers guidance on defining the population of American Indians and Alaska Natives for inclusion in a survey, enhancing participation of the tribes, and obtaining approval from the institutional review board; in addition, it discusses issues of confidentiality and anonymity of individuals and tribes.

Piquemal, N. (2001). Free and informed consent in research involving Native American communities. *░░eri░an ░ndian ░ulture and ░e░ear░░ ░░urnal░░*(1), 65–79.

> This article offers recommendations for negotiating responsibilities before seeking consent, obtaining consent from relevant authorities, reconfirming consent as work proceeds, and providing the community with data.

9.░ ░nal░░i░an░ ░ep░rting

Americans for Nonsmokers' Rights. (2007). *State░and ░uni░░alitie░░it░░░░░ ░░░░e░ree la░░in ░░r░░a░e░░re░░aurant░░░░ ░ar░* Retrieved February 6, 2009, from http://www.no-smoke.org/pdf/100ordlist.pdf

American Nonsmokers' Rights Foundation (2010a). *░░eri░an░░░r n░h░░░░░er░ rig░t░░ S░░░e░ree li░░░░░a░░░and data*. Retrieved June 8, 2010, from http://no-smoke.org/goingsmokefree.php?id=519

American Nonsmokers' Rights Foundation (2010b). *░░eri░an░░░r n░h░░░░░er░ rig░t░* Retrieved June 8, 2010, from http://no-smoke.org/index.php

American Nonsmokers' Rights Foundation (2010c). *░vervie░ li░t—░░░░ ░any ░░░░e░ree la░░░*Retrieved June 9, 2010, from http://www.no-smoke.org/pdf/mediaordlist.pdf

Anchorage voters embrace smoking ban (2007, April 7). *░h░░░░age ░aily ░e░░*

Biemer, P. P., & Lyberg, L. E. (2003). *░ntr░du░ti░n t░░urvey ░uality*. Hoboken, NJ: Wiley.

> This book is a nontechnical, comprehensive introduction to survey concepts, terminology, notation, and models.

Bondura, A. (1977). Self-efficacy: Toward a unifying theory of behavioral change. *P░y░░░░gi░al ░evie░░░░*, 191–215.

> This article is about the stages-of-change model.

Brownson, R. C., Hopkins, D. P., & Wakefield, M. A. (2002). Effects of smoking restrictions in the workplace. *░hnual ░evie░ ░░Pu░░i░░ealt░░░░*, 333–348.

Centers for Disease Control and Prevention. (1990). *░░e ░ealt░░ene░░░░░░░░ng ░e░░ati░n░░re░░░t ░░t░e Surge░n ░eneral*. Rockville, MD: Author.

Centers for Disease Control and Prevention. (1998). *░░░a░░░u░e a░░ng ░S░ra░░al░et░ni░ ░in░rity gr░u░░—░░i░an ░░eri░an░░░eri░an ░ndian░and ░a░░a ░ative░░░░░an ░░eri░an░and Pa░░░░░lander░░and ░░░ani░░░░re░░░t ░░t░e Surge░n ░eneral*. Atlanta, GA: Author.

Centers for Disease Control and Prevention. (2006). *░░e ░ealt░░░h░e░░uen░e░░░░nv░luntary e░░░░░ure t░t░░a░░░░░░░e░░re░░░t ░░t░e Surge░n ░eneral*. Atlanta, GA: Author.

Centers for Disease Control and Prevention. (2010). Tobacco Control State Highlights: Alaska. *S░░░ng and ░░░a░░░░░e*. Retrieved July 29, 2010, from http://www.cdc.gov/tobacco/data_statistics/state_data/state_highlights/2010/states/alaska/index.htm

DiClemente, C. C., Prochaska, J. O., & Gibertini, M. (1985). Self-efficacy and the stages of self-change in smoking. *░░gnitive ░░era░y and ░e░░ar░░░░*, 181–200.

> This article is about the stages-of-change model.

Doolan, D. M., & Froelicher, E. S. (2006). Efficacy of smoking cessation intervention among special populations: Review of the literature from 2000 to 2005. *Nursing Research*, *□*(4 Suppl.), S29–S37.

This article reviews the literature on smoking cessation among special populations, including American Indians and Alaska Natives.

Eichner, J. E., Cravatt, K., Beebe, L. A., Blevins, K. S., Stoddart, M. L., Bursac, Z., et al. (2005). Tobacco use among American Indians in Oklahoma: An epidemiologic view. *Public Health Reports*, *□*(2), 192–199.

This article compares tobacco-use findings from four major surveys of American Indians in Oklahoma in the 1990s.

Fleiss, J. L., Levin, B., & Paik, M. C. (2003). *Statistical methods for rates and proportions*. New York: Wiley.

Horwath, C. C. (1999). Applying the transtheoretical model to eating behavior change: Challenges and opportunities. *Nutrition Research Reviews*, *□*, 281–317.

This article is about the stages-of-change model.

Lohr, S. L. (1999). *Sampling: Design and analysis*. Pacific Grove, CA: Duxbury Press.

This book covers techniques for survey design and data analysis.

Mowery, P. D., Farrelly, M. C., Haviland, M. L., Gable, J. M., & Wells, H. E. (2004). Progression to established smoking among U.S. youths. *American Journal of Public Health*, *□*(2), 331–337.

National Cancer Institute (2010). *Tobacco use supplement to the current population survey (TUS-CPS) for tobacco monitoring and methods*. Retrieved June 8, 2010.

Nazaroff, W. W., & Singer, B. C. (2004). Inhalation of hazardous air pollutants from environmental tobacco smoke in U.S. residences. *Journal of Exposure Analysis and Environmental Epidemiology*, *□*(Suppl. 1), S71–S77.

Oswald, J. (2000). Minnesota Center for Excellence in Health Statistics. In *Proceedings of the Section on Survey Research Methods, American Statistical Association*. Alexandria, VA: American Statistical Association.

This paper reviews analytic methods to clarify public health issues related to minority population health disparities.

Pirkle, J. L., Flegal, K. M., Bernert, J. T., Brody, D. J., Etzel, R. A., & Maurer, K. R. (1996). Exposure of the U.S. population to environmental tobacco smoke: The Third National Health and Nutrition Examination Survey, 1988 to 1991. *Journal of the American Medical Association*, *□*(16), 1233–1240.

Pleninger, D., & Volk, T. (2005). *Puffballus lignarius used by native Americans with tobacco*. La Crosse: University of Wisconsin–La Crosse.

Prochaska, J. O., Velicer, W. F., DiClemente, C. C., & Fava, J. (1988). Measuring processes of change: Applications to the cessation of smoking. *Journal of Consulting and Clinical Psychology*, *□*, 520–528.

This article is about the stages-of-change model.

Prochaska, J. O., Velicer, W. F., Rossi, J. S., Goldstein, M. G., Marcus, B. H., Rakowski, W., et al. (1994). Stages of change and decisional balance for 12 problem behaviors. *Healt Psychology 13*, 39–46.

This article is about the stages-of-change model.

Shavers, V. L., Lawrence, D., Fagan, P., & Gibson, J. T. (2005). Racial/ethnic variation in cigarette smoking among the civilian U.S. population by occupation and industry, TUS-CPS 1998–1999. *Preventive Medicine 41*(2), 597–606.

This article is an examination of racial/ethnic variation in the prevalence of current smoking and cigarette consumption patterns by occupation, industry, and workplace smoking policy; it uses TUS-CPS data.

Shopland, D. R., Anderson, C. M., Burns, D. M., & Gerlach, K. K. (2004). Disparities in smoke-free workplace policies among food service workers. *Journal of Occupational and Environmental Medicine 46*(4), 347–356.

Tauras, J. A. (2007). Differential impact of state tobacco control policies among race and ethnic groups. *Addiction 102*(Suppl. 2), 95–103.

This article reviews patterns of racial and ethnic cigarette use in the United States and discusses changes in state-level tobacco control policies.

U.S. Census Bureau. (2008). *Current Population Survey (CPS): A joint effort by the Bureau of Labor Statistics and the Census Bureau*. Retrieved February 24, 2009, from www.bls.census.gov/cps/cpsmain.htm

Waksberg, J., Levine, D., & Marker, D. (2000). *Assessment of major federal data sets for analyses of Hispanic and Asian or Pacific Islander subgroups and Native Americans: Extending the utility of federal data bases*. Washington, DC: U.S. Department of Health and Human Services, Office of the Assistant Secretary for Planning and Evaluation.

This report offers a review of databases useful for comparison with data from the AN ATS.

Wasser, T. (2004). *A retrospective approach to design making for conducting public health interventions*. Paper presented at the Section on Health Policy Statistics, Joint Meeting of the American Statistical Association, Toronto, Ontario, Canada.

This paper offers methods for evaluation of community health interventions.

9.0 Program Planning

Alaska Department of Health and Social Services. (2004). *Tobacco in the great land: A portrait of Alaska's leading cause of death*. Retrieved February 24, 2009, from www.epi.hss.state.ak.us/pubs/tobaccofeb04.pdf

Alaska Department of Health and Social Services. (2006). Alaska tobacco facts. Retrieved July 7, 2010, from www.hss.state.ak.us/dph/chronic/tobacco/alaska_tobacco_facts.pdf

Alaska Department of Health and Social Services. (2006). Tobacco prevention and control in Alaska: Preventing addiction—Saving lives. Retrieved February 24, 2009, from http://www.hss.state.ak.us/dph/chronic/tobacco/ATCA_AR05.pdf

Alaska Department of Health and Social Services. (2007, March). *What state survey tell us about tobacco use among Alaska Native population: tobacco program planning executive summary*. Retrieved February 14, 2009, from www.hss.state.ak.us/dph/chronic/tobacco

Alaska Native Health Board. (n.d.). *Alaska Native Health Board*. Retrieved February 24, 2009, from www.anhb.org

Alaska Tobacco Control Alliance. (n.d.). *Alaska Tobacco Control Alliance: Creating conditions for Alaskans to live free from the harmful effects of tobacco*. Retrieved February 24, 2009, from www.alaskatca.org

Alaska Tobacco Quit Line, 1-888-842-QUIT (7848).

Center for Disease Control and Prevention. (2009). *Guide to community preventive services*. Retrieved February 24, 2009, from www.thecommunityguide.org

Centers for Disease Control and Prevention. (2008). *Smoking and tobacco use*. Retrieved February 24, 2009, from www.cdc.gov/tobacco

King, T. K., Borrelli, B., Black, C., Pinto, B. M., & Marcus, B. H. (1997). Minority women and tobacco: Implications for smoking cessation interventions. *Annal of Behavioral Medicine*, (3), 301–313.

> This article reviews the smoking behaviors of African American, American Indian and Native Alaskan, Asian and Pacific Islander, and Hispanic women smokers to develop strategies for smoking cessation treatment.

National Cancer Institute. (2009). Risk factor monitoring and methods: Tobacco use supplement. Retrieved February 24, 2009, from http://riskfactor.cancer.gov/studies/tus-cps/

State of Alaska Health and Social Services. (n.d.). Alaska Tobacco Prevention and Control Program. Retrieved February 24, 2009, from www.hss.state.ak.us/dph/chronic/tobacco

U.S. Census Bureau. (2001–2007). Tobacco Use Supplement, Current Population Survey [Data files]. *National Cancer Institute risk factor monitoring and methods website*. Retrieved February 24, 2009, from http://riskfactor.cancer.gov/studies/tus-cps/info.html

U.S. Census Bureau. (2008). *Current Population Survey (CPS): A joint effort by the Bureau of Labor Statistics and the Census Bureau*. Retrieved February 24, 2009, from www.bls.census.gov/cps/cpsmain.htm

U.S. Department of Health and Human Services. (2008). Protecting human research subjects: Institutional Review Board guidebook (S/N: 017-040-00525-3). Retrieved from www.hhs.gov/ohrp/irb/irb_guidebook.htm

www.ingramcontent.com/pod-product-compliance
Lightning Source LLC
Chambersburg PA
CBHW080308180526
45167CB00006B/2725